T0146647

PANNING FOR YOUR CLIENT'S GOLD

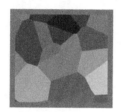

PANNING FOR YOUR CLIENT'S GOLD

12 Lean Clean Language Processes

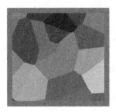

Gina Campbell

Balboa Press books may be ordered through booksellers or by contacting:

Balboa Press
A Division of Hay House
1663 Liberty Drive
Bloomington, IN 47403
www.balboapress.com
1 (877) 407-4847

Book layout design and typesetting by Amy Kopperude.
Cover design by Kendall Ludwig.

ISBN: 978-1-5043-2927-9 (sc)
ISBN: 978-1-5043-2928-6 (e)

Print information available on the last page.

Balboa Press rev. date: 6/2/2015

BALBOA.
PRESS
A DIVISION OF HAY HOUSE

Acknowledgments

Most of the Clean processes described in this book were conceived by counseling psychologist David Grove (1950–2008), the originator of Clean Language. Building on the basic Clean Language concepts developed by Grove and psychotherapist Cei Davies Linn, other processes herein were developed by James Lawley and Penny Tompkins. Emergent Knowledge coaching processes were developed by Grove with Clean coach Carol Wilson. The group metaphor process was based on a methodology developed by Caitlin Walker with additional input from James Lawley. When you have a group of people as creative, experimental, and generous as the Clean community members are in their sharing of ideas, it is difficult sometimes to know what started where. I have in all cases attributed ideas to their originators to the best of my knowledge and apologize to anyone whom I have inadvertently left unacknowledged.

My thanks to Penny Tompkins and James Lawley, to Wendy Sullivan, and to Angela Dunbar for introducing me to these techniques in trainings. Thanks also to EAGALA equine therapist Patti Schlough and equine specialist Michele Schraff for sharing with me their creative experiments with mixing and matching various Clean processes in their therapeutic work with clients and horses. Our brainstorming sessions and your facilitations are inspirational.

For their detailed reading and suggestions, thanks to Jill Rowan and, again and always, Penny Tompkins and James Lawley. What will hopefully read as an accurate book with a well-organized and logical flow involves months of hard work, revisions, and a thousand and one decisions. Having critical eyes and insightful suggestions was invaluable.

Note: You will notice I have opted to use the pronoun *he* most of the time when referring to clients or facilitators in general. This is out of frustration more than preference. It simply becomes unwieldy to have so many *she/he* and *his/her* pronouns. The former English teacher in me rails against using the plural pronoun *their* for the singular his or hers. And jumping back and forth between *he* and *she* from paragraph to paragraph or page to page is distracting. So I have opted for *he* to stand for all of us, as much as it hurts my feminist heart. Until English comes up with a genderless single pronoun or *their* becomes officially both plural and singular (as most of us use it when speaking), I will settle for this, with apologies to those who are sensitive to its implied inequality. I use both male and female clients in examples.

Welcome

Welcome, helping and healing professionals. If you are looking for creative yet simple ways to help your clients get transformational results, this book will introduce you to 12. These processes are designed to access your clients' subconscious mind/body system in ways that help your clients learn about themselves: to grow, to heal, to imagine, and to embrace new possibilities. They were developed by psychotherapist and master innovator David Grove and those who have followed in his giant footsteps.

Grove's work in the 1980s and 1990s was largely about working with clients' internal metaphors using his metaphor therapy and Clean Language processes. By 2002, he was exploring new ways to encourage a client to grow and heal with a greater emphasis on applying the principles of emergence. While this book includes some aspects of Grove's early work, it is largely about his work from 2000 through 2008 and what he called Emergent Knowledge processes.

The gift of time

How often do we give our clients the opportunity to spend uninterrupted time exploring what they know about a topic? Often we distract them by asking them to explain themselves, to listen to our well-intended but often diverting contributions, or to address what *we* decide is of importance. Even if they are given ample time for reflection, what with all the multitasking the modern world demands, many people have trouble sustaining their attention long enough to explore anything deeply.

While a few of these Clean processes are basically setups for a session, the majority of them offer your clients a chance to stay focused on one issue for an extended period of time. As you hold the space with Clean Language questions, your clients will discover much they don't yet know they know.

What attracts helping and healing professionals to use these lean Clean processes?

- Their *simplicity*: They are easy to learn and easy to apply.
- Their *experiential nature*: They engage clients in actively exploring themselves.
- Their *flexibility*: They can be used to assess and work on a wide variety of issues.
- Their *rapidity*: Clients connect to new and helpful experiences and insights quickly.
- Their *light touch*: While the client does not go deeply into any one memory, emotion, or issue, the processes can have a surprisingly powerful impact.

What follows is a description of *some* of the concerns and goals various types of helping professionals may have that these Clean processes can address. As there are overlaps between professions, I encourage you to read through them all to get ideas about what working with a Grovian Clean process could do for your clients, whatever your profession.

Perhaps you are a *counselor* or *therapist* who…

1. Wants an assessment of your clients' key issues to get a fuller picture than discussion about their presenting problems might offer. And you want to avoid getting buried under a mound of details that may not be relevant to the underlying issues. You want to get a broad overview quickly, efficiently, effectively, and respectfully in a way that accesses and honors your clients' deepest knowing.

2. Works with traumatized or anxious clients for whom going too deeply too quickly could be overwhelming. You want to avoid re-traumatizing them. You seek processes that help your clients explore their subconscious but in a way that allows them to have some distance from emotional issues and a feeling of being in control of the process so it feels safe.

3. Wants processes that keep your own assumptions and biases out of your clients' content.

4. Wants to help your clients learn to access and trust their intuitive knowing, a knowing that comes from a deeper place than talk generally reaches.

Perhaps you are a *career counselor, school counselor,* or *other professional* who…

1. Seeks to help clients clarify their values, interests, needs, goals, and priorities.

2. Wants activities your clients can do in just a portion of a session that will nevertheless give them access to profoundly relevant but rarely uncovered information about themselves.

3. Wants processes simple enough that your clients can learn to do them for themselves as future needs arise.

Maybe you are a *coach* who…

1. Wants to empower your clients to discover their own expertise and motivation.

2. Wants clear, structured models for helping your clients get clarity on their goals and their strategies for reaching them.

3. Wants to connect with your clients' relevant core issues without getting deeply into past history and therapeutic territory.

Or you are a *workshop leader* who…

1. Wants to facilitate people to get to know themselves better.

2. Works with groups and wants simple yet engaging activities that will help participants get to know and understand one another better.

3. Needs wording general enough that it can be used to guide a group session while allowing each person to explore what comes up for him personally.

4. Wants a group process that can improve communication and understanding between members and foster better team functioning.

The lean, Clean processes in this book can meet all of these needs and more. To fully appreciate their potential, I encourage you to experience as many of them as possible as a client. You could do this during a training with me or another Clean trainer, with a study buddy who's taking this journey with you, with a friend or family member who will read the scripts for you, or by experiencing a sample session with a trained Clean facilitator. You will discover that the answers you get to these deceptively simple questions come from a different place than information does in ordinary conversation.

Whatever kind of helping or healing professional you are, I am confident you will find ideas here to stimulate your thinking about how you can help foster your clients' self-exploration, growth, and healing. Try a few of these processes, and I am confident you will want to master them all for their rich potential.

Gina Campbell

Contents

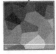

About This Book

What is *Clean* about these processes?

We will be considering Clean Language and the term Clean as Grove used it in much more detail later, but as you will come across both early on, let me explain ever so briefly what each one means.

To be Clean, according to Grove's concept, means the facilitator directs his client's attention among the words, images, and actions of that client. The facilitator avoids "dirtying" the client's content or his discovery and learning process with the facilitator's assumptions, interpretations, or advice; even his preferred word choices and metaphors are excluded during the Clean session. By sticking to the content the client introduces, the facilitator is assured of working from the client's model of his world.

To direct attention in a Clean way, the Clean facilitator uses a very limited number of simply worded questions and directives—called Clean Language—and the client's *exact* words.

What is *lean* about these processes?

In the later 1990s, David Grove began experimenting with new processes using Clean Language to address two goals. He wanted the processes to (1) be simple to learn and facilitate and (2) help a client glean helpful information from his subconscious world without getting deeply into it.

The processes in this book are generally brief and easy to learn and use with clients, so I call them *lean*. They are straightforward enough that with a practice round or two, you will be able to conduct a session using them. Though the processes are simple, that doesn't mean your client can't get a great deal of benefit from them. Prepare to be surprised.

To make it easy for you to learn 12 processes, I have in some instances tweaked Grove's wording of Clean questions to keep them more consistent from process to process. Grove often experimented with exact wording options for years, adding a word here, changing a word there, ever attuned to subtle nuances and playing with new ideas. We were left at Grove's sudden death with versions of Clean questions and directives he may well have continued to adjust. He also tweaked questions depending on the client in front of him, on what exactly he said. Not surprisingly then, I find different writers on Clean use slightly different phrasing variations. Given this history, I feel comfortable with limiting variations in wording to give you fewer phrases to master.

I also attempt to be lean when it comes to my explanations. There are other authors, whose articles and books you will find listed in the Bibliography and Endnote sections, who will give you more exhaustive Clean theory and its history and contributory concepts. I wrote this book for people who want to cut to the chase. If you are a practical person who prefers examples over in-depth explanations, you may find this a relief; but please, don't skip Section 1: Theories and Intentions. You are much more likely to use the processes *cleanly* and facilitate them well with some understanding of what's behind them. In addition, the section includes some important tips on facilitation techniques.

Why 12 processes?

David Grove, the developer of Clean Language and many subsequent Clean processes, was a great experimenter, full of creative ideas. This book includes processes that have caught on with the international Clean community and ones that I find I most often use with clients. There is plenty here to keep you busy discovering new ways to access your clients' inner world. And when you are ready for more, you can move on to my pair of workbooks on Clean Language and Symbolic Modeling[1] (Campbell, 2012, 2013).

This book's organization

Take a moment to look over the Contents page. After a general introduction, you will see that Sections 2 through 5 and Section 7 introduce the 12 processes in groups:

Section 2: Processes for getting a session off to a focused start

Section 3: Processes that have clients moving in space

Section 4: Processes that have clients writing or drawing on paper

Section 5: Processes for developing action plans

Section 7: Processes for group facilitating

Section 6 gives you some suggestions for segueing out of a Clean session *cleanly* and smoothly.

And finally, Section 8 will challenge you to be agile and creative with combining and applying processes.

Mixing media

You will notice in Section 8 that the processes developed to be applied to *space* can also be tweaked to work with *written* or *drawn* responses and vice versa. So enjoy familiarizing yourself with the processes in all the sections, even if you plan on using only one medium.

Uses

Each process is introduced with a brief description of what it is designed to do and suggestions as to what you might use it for. *These lists are by no means exhaustive*; no doubt you will think of many other applications. The same is true of the lists in Section 8 of suggested methodologies with which you can integrate Clean questions and various populations or themes with which you can use Clean processes.

Session examples

Examples of client sessions with typical responses are provided for every process, though some are abbreviated in the interest of keeping this book concise.

Scripts

At the end of the text you will find scripts for each of the processes described. Each script of directives and questions has been condensed to one page so that you can easily copy it and have it as a guide when you facilitate a session with your client. Once you master these basics, you may want to refer back to the detailed description of the process for some optional questions you can add.

Ways to use this book

This is a book to return to again and again; it is not meant to be digested all in one fell swoop. Once you have read the introductory section that gives you key concepts behind Clean processes and some facilitation directives, you could conceivably use this book by dipping in, grabbing one process to try with your clients, and coming back for more when you are ready. Or read through them all and see what captures your imagination or might best fit your context. There is an element of playfulness with all of the processes, a let's-see-what-happens openness about them that invites such experimentation.

The processes are ordered more or less in terms of complexity, with the simplest and shortest ones first. If you have experimented with the processes as you read along, by the time you get to Section 8, where I start blending questions from various processes, you are less likely to get overwhelmed at the idea of such mixing and matching. Then again, if you are the type of learner who likes to read everything through before actually trying out a new technique, by all means do so; just don't let this last section intimidate you. I wouldn't expect you to be able to do the sort of blending I demonstrate with client Matt, for example, without practice with the individual processes first.

The main message I want to convey to you is this: you have to actually *do* sessions. The difference between reading a book like this and finding it a "stimulating read" and having it rock your world is in the doing! Don't let perfectionism stop you. Clean sessions can still be very effective even with the occasional fumble, and it doesn't take long to get good with these simple processes.

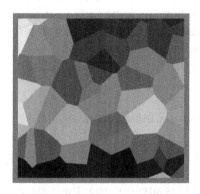

Theories
and Intentions

PANNING FOR YOUR CLIENT'S GOLD

If you are a miner and you want to find gold, there are two ways to go about it. You can mine it, going deep in the earth to search for veins of it. With luck, you tap a primary vein: "hit the mother lode," as they say. The other option is to pan for it, to sift the gravel carried by a stream through a sieve to find what are usually small nuggets. Chance upon a large nugget or find enough smaller ones, and you can amass a wealth of gold.

As a helping or healing professional, you can assist your client in finding his gold, that valuable material that enriches his life by bringing understanding, new perspectives, and sometimes significant shifts and healing. To find it, you could invite him to go deeply into his past and present issues and his mind/body system, like a miner. Or you can guide him to pan for it: you encourage information from the subconscious to come to the surface, touching upon it lightly and briefly. This allows the individual to find his own answers at his own pace, using his expertise on the intricacies of his own self and situation.

Panning for our clients' gold with Clean processes is about:

- Where we as facilitators direct our clients' attention to look for information
- How many and what questions we ask
- How long we spend asking about any one specific detail

Sometimes it benefits your client not to go deeply but to hold his attention near the surface and see what rises to it. This book will give you the right tools and skills to help that happen.

Before we get to the lean Clean processes themselves, let me introduce you to David Grove, the original thinker and grand experimenter who pushed the boundaries of counseling and coaching into new frontiers.

DAVID GROVE

David Grove (1950–2008), originally from New Zealand, was a counseling psychologist by training. Among his early interests in therapeutic techniques were NLP (neurolinguistic programming), Eriksonian hypnosis, and the works of Virginia Satir and Carl Rodgers. Observing and experimenting with clients from his psychotherapy practice, he went on to develop his own theories as to:

- How people internally or subconsciously structure their experiences
- What needs to happen for people to change
- Innovative counseling and coaching processes to help them do it

Most of the 12 Clean processes we will cover are Grove's. A few were developed by others using his general Clean questioning approach.

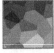

To give you a conceptual framework to understand what these processes are intended to achieve, let me briefly present six concepts that informed Grove's work. They do not build in a strictly sequential fashion, and there is some overlap. I invite you to notice the concepts' common ground and consider their reoccurring aspects from different perspectives.

But first…

THE SCIENCE OF EMERGENCE

Emergence attempts to explain how a collection of individual units become complex, self-directing systems.[2] From evolutionary leaps in nature to the growth of cities, from busy ant colonies to sensitive stock markets, self-organizing systems and patterns emerge from innumerable small interactions of the system's parts in response to simple guiding rules, repetitions, and feedback.

When a system reaches a level of complexity for which the existing management structure is no longer adequate, a transformation occurs. Something new, something that is more that just a sum of its parts, comes into existence. By definition, emergent features are unpredictable; there will be characteristics of the new whole that do not exist among its component parts. Thus you cannot know in advance what the "new" will be. Nor can you predict precisely if or when a shift will occur.

Shifts in organizational patterns sift down through the system. In a process termed *downward causation,* the original component parts that made up the system are affected by the new structure. They change because the individual's system has a feedback loop: it learns from itself. The parts are no longer exactly as they were before.

To give you an example of something that demonstrates emergence, think of a rioting mob. A collection of individuals gather, certain influences are brought to bear—perhaps a speaker inciting hate or a small but critical mass of those present start to run—and individuals start to behave en masse the way they would not alone, often without making a conscious decision to do so. What emerges is a mob mentality. To use a more positive example, take a group of athletes. Individually, they have skills, strengths, and weaknesses and may play a certain way, etc. But something happens to the individuals when they bond as a team. The coach will know it when it happens, for a team is something more than its individual players. It demonstrates a collective, higher order of functioning.

From the microlevel of quantum physics to the macrolevel of the global economy, there are multitudinous examples of emergence at all levels when conditions give rise to some new structure of organization. Fundamental to this concept is that the reorganizing of the system happens naturally, without needing a structural organizer from outside the system. Over the long term, the system self-regulates.

GUIDING CONCEPT #1: We are self-organizing, self-correcting systems

David Grove applied emergence theory to the individual, regarding him as a system of interrelating parts with numerous bits of information, experiences, and coping strategies accumulated over the years. At any given time the system has an organizing structure, a modus operandi or way of functioning.

When the individual has a problem, a contributing factor may be that his system's organization is not optimized to resolve it. Healthy or helpful functioning is not a result of *what* the interrelating parts are; it is a matter of organization, of *how* the parts are interacting, which is why, for example, two soldiers with similar combat experiences may experience very different long-term effects.

According to the principles of emergence, with enough pieces of information relating to the problem, a system with a less-than-optimal way of organizing that information will eventually find a better way. This new structure of organization leads to the clients' having a different way of coping or managing, which can in turn, mean new choices and outcomes are possible.

For some clients, the shift filters through the system's parts rapidly. The old structure may have proved to be so inadequate that it collapses and spontaneously disappears entirely. Other times, the new pattern of organization that emerges may incorporate some or all of the old pattern.

Still other times, the old pattern gradually fades away. Given our mind/body system's natural tendency to self-correct to function efficiently and beneficially, as the new structure demonstrates to the mind/body system its more beneficial, stable way of functioning, it becomes the go-to pattern of responding.

Depending on the pressures on it, the new emergent state exists for awhile (maybe for a very long while) until some new dilemma challenges it. This creates a pressure for change, and at some point, a new order will again emerge.

It is a dynamic process of self-correction.

So what might happen when a client's system reorganizes? Of course it is different for each individual, depending on what's needed. In terms of observable effects, I have had clients finally leave a job or relationship, change careers, decide to have an operation, start exercising regularly, lose weight, start AA, have a difficult conversation, cease debilitating grieving, forgive themselves, and do all sorts of things that they had agonized over for months, if not years. Sometimes the effects are more about a pervasive feeling: a sense of relief or joy or engagement with life. Their systems evolve a new coping strategy that allows them to establish a new modus operandi.

Suggestions that come from the outside, that is, any external source such as a therapist's or coach's ideas or solutions, may or may not penetrate to the system level; if they do, they may not override old patterns and beliefs.

David Grove maintained that comprehensive and lasting change, change that resonates throughout the individual's entire system, requires structural reorganizing from within.

How do Grovian processes apply emergence theory?

All Grovian processes rely on the characteristics of emergent systems to naturally self-correct, even those David Grove developed before he began to study the science of emergence specifically (Lawley & Tompkins, 2000). Grove's intention with Clean interventions was to *optimize the conditions* whereby the client discovers, accesses, and accumulates information from his mind/body system, including relevant data that may have been inaccessible or unrecognized before.

The processes focus the Clean facilitator on structuring the exploratory experience rather than introducing any new content.

Grove used the term *Emergent Knowledge* to describe his processes that most fully assign the job of identifying and exploring elements of his inner system to the client himself. In Emergent Knowledge processes, developed by Grove and Clean coach Carol Wilson, the facilitator follows a scripted sequence of questions and directives, giving the client's system full rein to determine what sort of information gets collected.

GUIDING CONCEPT #2: Work from the bottom up

Fundamental to the processes David Grove developed is the respect in which he held the client's wisdom and the confined role he assigned for the coach, therapist, or other helper or healer. In Clean processes the client, not the professional, is the expert on himself. The professional is there to hold the space and facilitate the client's exploration. Grove would surely never have assigned so little responsibility to the facilitator and so much to the client unless he truly believed—and had seen demonstrated quite literally thousands of times in his practice—that clients have within what they need to heal.

So if the client is to get accurate information about his inner organizing structure, where does the facilitator direct him to start looking?

Top-down approaches

Helping professionals using top-down approaches start with preestablished generalities, to which a client is compared. This might mean referring to a list of categories to which the client is matched. These categories then suggest appropriate ways to diagnose and work with the client. Examples would be the *DSM-V*, Enneagrams, and the Meyers-Briggs Inventory.

While some practitioners adhere to their chosen framework without deviance, others use the frameworks to inform, but not dictate, what they do. In either case, a top-down approach

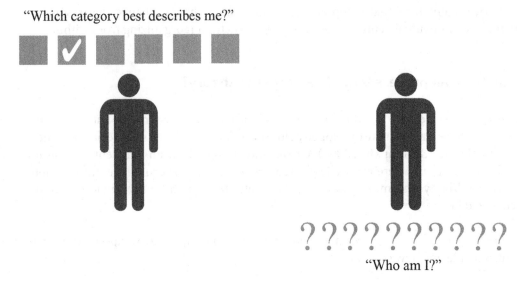

Top-down vs. bottom-up methodologies

inevitably involves applying some assumptions. If your framework has only square boxes, you will probably be looking for and asking about only what is in the square boxes. You risk missing entirely what's outside the boxes, *especially if your client isn't consciously aware of it.*

A bottom-up approach

Grove believed that to help a client learn about and help himself, he is best off working from the bottom up, that is, starting from scratch. No predetermined boxes. The facilitator encourages the client to expand his self-awareness by helping him find fundamental self-definitions: Who am I? What do I know? What do I want? What needs to change for me to get what I want? These are broad, generic questions that provide no implicit answers.

David Grove determined to make as few assumptions as possible in the way he worked. His guiding intention was to work with the client's own content only, trusting that the client would find for himself what he needs.

Equal information employers

One of the distinguishing characteristics of Grove's Clean processes is they are designed to work with whatever the client offers up, regardless of the kind or source of information. They are what Grove called "equal information employers." Information may come from the past or the present or be oriented to the future. It can be a feeling, a thought, a belief, a behavior, or a gesture. It can be an image, a metaphor, or a sound. Its relevance may not be immediately obvious to you or the client. But with patience and trust in the process and in the client, what is needed will emerge.

GUIDING CONCEPT #3: We learn best through experiences

You might be wondering: if emergence theory applies to individuals, if they are self-correcting and self-organizing, then why are so many people confused, dysfunctional, or otherwise not able to act in their own best interests? Because there's yet another key element of a responsive, self-correcting mind/body system. You can have identified the process—encouraging conditions for emergence leads to self-correction. You can know the source of the information needed for self-correction—the client. You can know from which direction to work—the bottom up. But you also have to be able to *access* the needed information.

How do you access relevant information, especially if it is subconscious?

When you work with Grovian processes, you come to realize that having your client spend a lot of time talking about what happened in his past or about his present is not as helpful as you might think (assuming, of course, we are not talking about someone who is in danger). Knowing a client's history, the *what* of his story, may not be all that relevant; often more important are questions about the *how*. How does his system function? What lessons for surviving and thriving has it learned? What coping strategies has it adopted? Do they serve him well? What internal resources does he rely on? How do any or all of these need to change?

It is the difference between focusing on the *content* of your client's history and the way he *processes* information, all types of information: mental, emotional, physical, behavioral, spiritual, internal, external, etc.

Experiential processes

Directly asking a client these *how* questions is not likely to be particularly revealing. Most of us don't have much insight into how we do what we do. Some of us are good at coming up with explanations if asked, for the human mind naturally seeks to create a narrative. But often it turns out our conscious, cognitive awareness is incomplete.

Our subconscious minds are much better sources for this how-I-do-it (or can't-do-it) sort of information. And the way to access the subconscious best is through experiential processes that engage the whole mind/body.

While early practitioners of experiential processes relied on experimenting and making qualitative assessments of the processes' effectiveness, recent research into how the brain works offers still another argument in their favor. For the brain to be receptive to learning and change, to exhibit what is termed *brain neuroplasticity,* the conditions that need to be met are the very ones that such processes create. As Daniel Seigel (2010), clinical professor of psychiatry at the UCLA School of Medicine and expert in the field of the relationship between brain science and psychotherapy, describes it:

> Under the right conditions, neural firing can lead to strengthening of synaptic connections. These conditions include repetition, emotional arousal, novelty, and the careful focus of attention. Strengthening synaptic linkages between neurons is how we learn from experience. (p. 40)

As you learn the Clean processes in this book and, hopefully, experience them yourself, I think you will find each of these criteria is met: the *repetition* of words and questions, the surprisingly *visceral and emotional* quality of the client's experience, the *novelty* of what I call "experiencing oneself" through metaphors and process-guided moving in space, and a slowing down and extended *careful focusing of attention*.

I would add that Grove studied hypnosis and deliberately designed Clean Language questions, with their unique wording and rhythm, to naturally induce a light trance state, from which the subconscious is more readily accessible.

As the client's brain is primed to be more flexible, more open to new learning and possibilities, he may be able to let disturbing or problematic neural connections fade. He may eject old patterns and establish new priorities, new responses, and new patterns. Engaged in an *experiential* process, the client's mind/body/brain system may more readily self-correct.

TAKING STOCK

So let's review for a moment.

Guiding Concept #1: People are systems that self-correct based on the principles of emergence.

Guiding Concept #2: To achieve an accurate model of his organizing structure, an individual should work from the bottom up.

Guiding Concept #3: We learn best and thus change most readily through "experiencing ourselves" by engaging in experiential processes that put us in touch with our subconscious understanding of how we do what we do.

So exactly what kind of experiential processes that use the principles of emergence and work from the bottom up reveal the building blocks of an individual's internal organizing structure? And how can we effectively increase the chances that neither the facilitator nor the facilitation process he uses interferes with the client's system of self-correction?

GUIDING CONCEPT #4: We encode our experiences in metaphors

Back in the 1980s, as David Grove worked with phobias and trauma, he came to believe that re-experiencing a traumatic event was neither cathartic nor beneficial. He determined to find ways to help his clients heal that did not risk re-traumatizing them.

It was at this time that Grove observed his clients' tendencies to use *metaphors* to describe how they felt or what something was like for them without having to actually talk about their fears, shame, or pain. Grove heard something that few other therapists and theorists had: he sensed there was more going on with these *client-generated* metaphors than their use for descriptive purposes. He explored what other role metaphors play in clients' mind/body system and experimented with how to work with them therapeutically. The conclusions he came to explain the radical departure his work took from that of Erickson, Satir, and others who used *therapist-provided* metaphors.

We will just scratch the surface of this work with metaphors with the use we make of it in the panning processes we will cover in this book. But here at least, are the basics of Grove's therapeutic metaphor theory so you will understand his reasoning behind his focus on internalized metaphors.

Before we dive in, let me offer a definition of metaphor.

> One thing is equated to a decidedly different thing in order to clarify the nature of the first thing's traits or qualities.

Often metaphors compare an abstract concept or feeling, such as loyalty or love, to something tangible, such as Velcro or an evergreen tree. Grove uses the term *metaphor* broadly; he included similes, analogies, parables, and the like.

Example

Client: *I've come to a fork in the road, and I have to decide which road I'm going to take.*

The client is not actually in front of two roads, of course, but the thoughts and/or feelings he has when he tries to make this particular choice are similar in his experience. No doubt you are familiar with such descriptions and use metaphors yourself.

When we use metaphors to better explain what something is like for us, aren't we just waxing poetic? Coming up with a catchy or elegant way of explaining ourselves? You may ask, what has it got to do with growth or healing?

Grove theorized that we all, consciously or subconsciously, encode our key experiences in metaphor. It is how we store them, filing similar experiences together under the heading of a metaphor that captures the essence of the experience or a key aspect of it. Common metaphors we can all probably relate to are:

It's like *hitting my head against a brick wall.*
Just thinking about doing that *gives me butterflies* in my stomach.
I'm not *getting into the middle of this.*
He's *got my back.*
Let me *take the wheel.*

While we may think we are simply using these metaphors descriptively, just ask a few simple questions, using any of the examples above, of any group of people who say they can relate to them from their own experiences. You will discover that there is a more specific meaning behind each one that is different for each person. What Grove found is, given a few of the *right kinds* of questions, you can find the details about the person's words and images that offer windows into his internal mind/body system, including his strategies for responding to a similar experience in the future.

When a challenging situation arises, the subconscious digs into its files to determine how to handle it. "How should I respond to keep safe? To be loved? To stay in control? To be congruent with my values?" Whatever the individual's internal system's goals are, he has strategies for achieving them based on past experience. And the medium in which these strategies are stored in the subconscious is metaphor. The metaphor may have been developed that morning or many years ago as a small child.

> Metaphors are like the genes of cells of the DNA—genetic codes that replicate. So if we want to change a repetitive or habitual experience, it's the replicating mechanism that matters…Find those structures so we can intervene at this level. It's different from trying to change the content. The content doesn't matter.[3]
>
> —David Grove

The metaphors may be described verbally (like the fork in the road). They might also be expressed with gestures/body language (a pushing away with the hand, a cringing of the shoulder) or as physical symptoms (a tightening in the gut, tension in the neck). The metaphors can be emotions or sensations (fear in the heart, calm in the breath). And they can be thoughts ("I'm not *up to* the task," "I *bring* a lot *to the table*").

Metaphors can support or thwart

Grovian processes are guided by the concept that these internalized metaphors, for better or for worse and *whether or not we are conscious of them,* frame how we think, feel, and behave. They can empower us or cripple us, support us or thwart us.

Fully embracing this concept of how the mind/body system functions in response to its metaphors has significant implications for working with clients. Grove developed Clean Language specifically to work with clients' internalized metaphors to effect healing and growth. The lean processes in this book focus on change that comes through greater awareness; often simply finding and getting familiar with his internalized metaphors is what a client needs for a new structure or organization to replace the old, less functional one.

During or after a session, a client often describes experiencing a "shift." Sometimes he can't say exactly what happened. Some of what gets activated in the client's system remains cloaked in the mystery of metaphor. He will report that he does not have to work at changing his feelings or behaviors; the new way is just "the way it is now." Something feels fundamentally and often profoundly different, and what was difficult before now seems "effortless."

Notice: Grove's processes use only the *client's* metaphors. You can give someone a metaphor to solve his dilemma, but yours may not land as deeply nor integrate into his system the way his own is integrated. And you risk leaving his own unresolved metaphors still inside to thwart his healing or growth. Offering your client suggestions for how to change his metaphors rather than letting him devise his own runs similar risks. More on this when we get to what being Clean is about in detail later in this section.

How do Grovian processes help a client access his internalized metaphors?

Often, a client will simply offer up his internalized metaphors when he is talking; they are, after all, the basic vocabulary his system uses. But if a client does not spontaneously offer a metaphor, it is surprisingly easy to help him access one, so much so that it is easy to undervalue Grove's contribution. You can do it with some careful listening and a few simple Clean Language questions that induce a sort of hypnotic, mindful inner focus. But I find the easiest ways for beginners to help a client find his metaphors are the ones you'll use with the 12 Clean processes in this book:

(1) Have him *draw* his answer to the Clean Language questions.

Anything short of an actual photographic likeness of an object is to some degree metaphoric. A picture's aim is to get some approximation of what something is *like*. And when it comes to depicting a feeling or abstract concept, what else can you use but a metaphor or symbol?

(2) Have him move about *in space* in response to Clean Language questions and directives.

If you project an inner experience into the space around you, it *will* include metaphoric information, as this next section makes clear.

GUIDING CONCEPT #5: We are fundamentally spatial beings

From the moment we are born (and arguably even before), we experience a sense of inside and outside. Just hours old, we have experienced a sense of things beneath us, above us, behind us, around us, and near and far. As we develop, we use this basic kinesthetic experience of the world to help make sense of what we think, feel, and otherwise experience. It comes as naturally to us to think and to communicate in spatial terms as to breathe because like the air, space is the medium in which we function.

Negotiating our way through the physical space around us is such an intrinsic part of this func-tioning that space-related concepts provide us with easily grasped metaphors to describe our experience of our world, often without even noticing we are doing it (Lakoff & Johnson, 1980).

Consider the following statements:

I need to *step back* and reconsider my decision.
I'm *getting ahead* of myself.
It's *out of my reach.*
I'm *beside myself* with worry!

Notice how in each example, there is an implied placing of the self in space. In some cases, there is a desire to change something about the self's location. Remarks like those above demonstrate that we organize our thinking and feelings by *locating* information.

Consider how we use space to describe time. For almost all cultures in the world, the future is described as being ahead, in the direction we naturally walk toward. The past is behind us, the space we leave if we are walking.

He's got a bright *future ahead* of him.
I *look forward* to getting together next week.
I'm glad that's *behind me* now.
Hold on a minute (as if you could stop time by holding onto it to keep it from moving).

So what does all this have to do with helping and healing people?

Grove's experiments confirmed that people not only use spatial language to describe their inner goings-on (they are, after all, metaphors). He also found that when clients move about in actual space, guided by a Clean process, they can discover much that they did not know they knew as they project their inner experience and knowing into the space around them.

Understanding that people can access bits of their inner wisdom by changing where they place themselves and that doing so can help disconnected parts of the self discover and learn from each other offers dazzling possibilities for working with people in new ways.

How do Grovian processes use space?

Grove developed numerous processes to encourage a client to explore an issue, problem, or goal by externalizing the relevant bits and parts of his subconscious, including its metaphors, out onto locations in a room or area or onto a piece of paper. Grove called a space that becomes imbued with such inner knowing of the client's mind/body *psychoactive*.

It is unexpected and truly remarkable to experience: as you stand in different spaces, you access different information. Choose a spot based on a Clean process directive or question, and information feels like it "downloads" into your awareness.

The processes are scripted and quite straightforward. They seem so simple that it is hard to believe as you read them that anything remarkable could happen. And yet, it does. Grove was on to something when he recognized the implications of our mind's fundamental spatial orientation.

GUIDING CONCEPT #6: Minimize contamination of the client's content

You may have noticed in the five guiding concepts above that not one of them suggests that the way to help a client depends on words, images, or solutions contributed by the facilitator. If we are, indeed, *self-organizing* systems, as Guiding concept #2 maintains, then the relevant "parts" to reorganize are the individual's. Grove embraced this concept wholeheartedly. He experimented for years to hone ways to help a client heal and grow without inadvertently inserting his own content. He wanted to work within the client's model of the world, honoring its own language and logic. He called this being *Clean*.

We are not talking about simple nondisclosure of personal information on the part of the therapist or coach. We are talking about structuring the facilitator's comments so that, for example, he makes no substitutions for the client's words that he *assumes* mean the same thing the client means. Grove's concern was that such redefining "robs the client of some of [his] experience."[4]

Beyond that still, we are talking about keeping out of the content of the session the facilitator's own metaphors—the ones he uses, consciously or subconsciously, to make sense of the world from *his* perspective. Since most of us are unaware of these metaphors and their influence, leaving it to the facilitator's conscious censoring, especially when he has so much else to be paying attention to, is unlikely to be successful. Grove's structured Clean questions do the censoring for the facilitator.

Other facilitators may tell you they don't lead clients, but once you examine the lengths Grovian processes go to to minimize the facilitator's word choices, the subtlety of Clean questions and directives and how they use the clients' exact words, you will soon notice that in comparison, others lead their clients much more than they may realize.

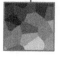

It is Grove's extraordinary sensitivity to and appreciation of the integrity of the client's experience—and the ways he found to respect it as he helps the client heal himself—that is his greatest legacy, I believe. Becoming a Clean facilitator means that you too will become more sensitized to whether you are working from your client's domain or your own. Your heightened awareness will better enable you to choose from which to work.

Giving advice

What about the client who wants advice? Begs for it? Will go to someone else to get it? What about clients who expect your expertise and input? Isn't that part of your role?

Your contract will vary depending on whether you are a life coach, a counselor or therapist, a workshop leader, etc. But whatever the situation, consider this:

> Your client is the expert on himself.
> True empowerment comes from finding the answers for oneself.

No matter how good your advice is, it may not be as helpful as you think.

- Clients are not always that perceptive about what the underlying issues of a problem are. You can end up putting a lot of time, attention, and energy into addressing the wrong issue when you address their plea for advice.

- Just because you give advice doesn't mean a client will follow it.

- If your advice proves unhelpful, the effects may go beyond its immediate impact. For example, rather than take responsibility for his choices, your client could blame you. Or he may swear off getting professional help in the future, needed though it may be. A failure may deplete his motivation to change. And following your advice could make the situation worse or cause new, unanticipated problems. No doubt you can think of more potential problems.

- You encourage your client's dependence on you.

Which is why, if your clients do not know how to access their inner organization and wisdom and do not have a clear sense of their own strengths, learning *how* to connect with them could be as valuable as the answers themselves.

Now, I am not saying there is no place for giving information. But there is a difference between providing *information,* such as what constitutes good nutrition, and giving *advice,* such as what to say to yourself to manage a strong temptation to overeat. What I am talking about avoiding is the latter. Internalized self-talk and strategies are better left to the individual to devise for himself in most cases.

Reframing

When I was in a counseling program in graduate school, professors encouraged me to help a client by offering a reframe. Essentially, I was to repeat my client's statements but use my own words. Not only was this meant to assure my client that I had listened to and understood him, but I could use this review as an opportunity to use my version of what my client said to suggest a different way of perceiving his situation or responses to it, a way that would lead my client to think, feel, and/or act in a healthier or more helpful way in regard to it.

Sounds good on the face of it, but if I want my client to get the most out of his sessions with me, this cognitive reframing requires that I know my client and his situation so well, with all its nuances and complexity, that I will offer the most appropriate perspective and solution for my client at that moment.

No matter how much experience I may have with clients with similar issues, just how much of an expert can I be when it comes to *this* individual? Can I ever know him as well as he knows himself?

The problem with reframing is, it is rife with assumptions. That what I have heard from him is accurate and comprehensive. That I know what my client means by the words he chooses. That he will readily correct me if I get it wrong; that he is not inclined to agree with my restatement out of embarrassment, confusion, a desire to cooperate, or confidence that as the expert, I must be right (to name but a few possibilities). That my suggestion takes into account all his context; that I can adequately incorporate his cultural, generational, gender, or other possible differences from me. And on and on and on.

Useful discipline

But, you say, your clients have often told you your reframe was so helpful! And I don't doubt it was. Sometimes a client can use and integrate your suggestion. But was it actually needed? And was it the best way to help? And was it given at the optimal time?

Often helping and healing professionals offer up their own advice before the client has had a chance to fully explore his issue for himself and before he has revealed much of what can inform the professional's interjection. Following a Clean process not only helps the client discover his inner self; it holds the facilitator back to allow subconscious content the time and space to reveal itself. The client may come up with his own reframe—an emergent reorganization of sorts.

When I am facilitating a Clean process, I feel again and again the discipline it instills in me. I am reminded each time a session takes a turn that surprises me that I might have led my client in a another direction had I intervened and he might have missed this piece of his puzzle. For most clients in most situations, my reframes are not needed. I would just distract my client by giving suggestions to be analyzed, weighed and then resisted, rejected, or accepted. Instead, my client works it out for himself from within the context of his own inner reality.

Encouraging self-exploration

With lean Clean processes, your role is primarily to hold the space and ask the scripted questions in a manner that encourages self-exploration. You are there to slow your client down and extend his attention on his topic and, particularly, on information about it that comes from his subconscious. You help hold his attention there long enough for him to discover his unseen "gold."

As your client discovers more of his own wisdom and expands his own worldview:

- He will internalize much more about how to approach a similar problem in the future.

- He may uncover other related issues neither of you may have known about or have considered.

- He will come up with solutions tailor-made for his situation.

- He will feel empowered by having done it for himself.

The intent to stay out of a client's content as much as possible is why I like the term "facilitator." To facilitate means to make easier; your role is to facilitate your client's accessing of his inner world and work with and through what emerges.

A paradigm shift

If that is not the way you have been working, you may seriously question such an approach. As counselors, therapists, coaches, workshop leaders, etc., with all our training, experience, and gifts, we no doubt have useful insights to offer clients. But give clients a chance and it turns out they are actually surprisingly good at discovering for themselves what it is they need once you help them access the whole of their knowing, their full mind/body wisdom. And that is what these experiential processes do.

I think of Clean processes as encouraging *self-exploration* rather than *self-explanation*. The client does not need to explain himself; he does not need to devote multiple sessions to filling you in on things he already knows. He does not need to revisit and recount his story. He can immediately begin exploring what more he needs to know and experience to foster the clarity and change he seeks.

Because the client is determining the content and to a large degree controls what is explored and the pace at which discoveries and change happen, a Clean session is empowering. Even after the session is over, the client retains the experience of having been the expert on himself. The Clean process deeply honors his knowing.

In fact, you could conduct an entire Clean session and not know what the client's subject of exploration is. You can invite your client to give the topic a name or label by which you will refer to it when facilitating, and he can keep his answers entirely unspoken. Personally, I do not tend to work like this, and my clients are not generally interested in it. But it is quite possible. Imagine the respect that conveys! The message you are sending is, "I have the tools to help you explore this, but the wisdom you discover is all coming from you."
Do you question whether you can help a person if you are in the dark? The naked truth is, regardless of the methodology we use, what we know about our clients is never entirely accurate or complete. While we have glimpses of their inner worlds, they will never be totally revealed to us. We always work from a place of limited knowing.

If this Clean philosophy requires a paradigm shift on your part, I invite you to open yourself to exploring a different way of thinking and working, whether you will ultimately choose to integrate Clean processes and/or questions selectively with what you already do or embrace it with all you do.

Having completed our review of six guiding concepts, I trust you have a basic sense now of *what* it is Clean processes are intended to do and *why*. We turn our attention now to *how*.

CLEAN LANGUAGE

It was the 1980s when David Grove first developed his metaphor therapy and Clean facilitating concepts. His Clean Language evolved as a tool to effectively (1) encourage his clients' experiential self-exploration, particularly of internalized metaphors, and (2) keep the facilitator's language, metaphors, assumptions, and worldview out of his client's content. Grove crafted deliberately short and simple questions. With carefully selected wording, syntax (the particular arrangement of the words), and rhythm, they ask for details of the client's *exact* words.

What is a Clean Language question?

The characteristics of a Clean Language question (CLQ) follow:

- It uses simple words. To paraphrase Grove, people are complex, so let the process and words you use to facilitate them be simple. The goal is not to engage the client cognitively but to ask questions of a deeper place; we aim not just for the brain but also for the heart, gut, throat, and whatever other parts speak up when the client looks for answers.

- The facilitator adds no words of his own beyond the simple words of the CLQ. Not a little phrase here, a compliment or encouraging word there. NONE! If the facilitator uses any other words besides those in the Clean question, it is only to repeat the client's exact words.

- Grovian processes use a limited number of questions that are repeated exactly, using the same wording with little variation. For the more questions you use and the more variations you add, the more time and attention your client has to put toward noting and making sense of them. What happens when you use a few simple questions over and over is that they become so predictable that the client doesn't need to expend much processing effort; in fact, after the session, he may say that he sort of forgot you were even there. Good! That means he was totally absorbed in his own world and did not find you intrusive.

- It may be somewhat awkward grammatically and have a distinct rhythmic quality. I have come to appreciate the value of CLQs not sounding like ordinary conversation, because that is exactly what you want to signal to your client: we are not having a conversation here. This is about your client's exploring his inner world for himself, not his telling you about it. And the distinct grammar and rhythm enhance the question's hypnotic effect.

  Grove described his CLQs as "very trance inducing without an induction. It is a natural induction because the questions do not pull the client out of his *experience*"[5] (italics added). The intention of a Clean question is to avoid having the client run the question through his "normal cognitive process" and stay tapped into what clients often describe as their deeper knowing. (In some contexts where a hypnotic state would not be appropriate, you may want to use more conversational wording. We will get to that in Section 8: Conversational Clean questions.)

- It starts with the word "And…". Starting a sentence with "And…" gives it a rhythmic cadence and helps get your client into and to stay in that mindful, inner-focused state. It serves as a repeated reminder that this is a special sort of experience, not a regular conversation. At least in my experience as a client, the "And…" subtly suggests my facilitator is just picking up on my last thought and following on through to the next. It suggests too that there is a next thought. And because the content of those thoughts is entirely mine, I almost stop noticing he is even there. The facilitator is situated, both literally and figuratively, on the periphery of my experience. (Grove included the "And…" deliberately for its trance-inducing influence. If you are working in a context where that mindful, trancelike focus is not appropriate, you may want to leave out the "And…".)

- It is for your client's benefit, not yours. A Clean question is selected to direct the client's attention to learn more about some particular of his that will help clarify and expand what he knows about himself and his inner world. It is not so that you, the facilitator, can understand more about the client. Rest assured, both you and your client *will* learn more about the many moving parts of his system related to some issue, but what you glean will be a byproduct of the session, not its driving force. That said, these Clean processes make excellent assessment tools.

You will be introduced to a number of CLQs in this book, but to give you an idea of what I mean by the six characteristics above, here are a few examples (the bold words are the standard questions, and the regular font identifies the client's exact words).

Client: *I feel a relaxation in my gut.*

Facilitator: **And is there anything else about that** relaxation in your gut?

               And what do you know now...about relaxation?

               And what kind of relaxation **is that** relaxation?

Clean directives

You will notice in the 12 processes covered here that there are several Clean directives; the statements may direct a client to "find" or "put down" for example. While they are not questions, they have characteristics similar to those of CLQs and should be repeated precisely, as with all Clean questions.

FACILITATING TIPS

We are almost ready to begin exploring Grove's Clean processes. But first, I would like to make some suggestions regarding how you facilitate a Clean session because it is different from what you are likely used to doing. Take the time to read and sit with the following concepts. And when you start practicing, explain them briefly to your practice buddy and ask him to give you some feedback on how you are doing.

Facilitating skills are a VERY big part of what makes these processes effective.

Preparing your client

Because these processes often put you in a role that a client may not expect from a therapist, counselor, coach, etc., you may want to spend some time thinking about how you will introduce them to your client before you begin. As you invite your client to focus in a mindful way on his inner experience and consult his intuitive sense, you will not want his concentration interrupted by needing to ask for explanations.

Consider discussing:

- Your role: Let your client know this is not about having a conversation with you. You will be asking him to identify and move to various locations in the space or asking some simple questions to direct his attention to various parts of a drawing. He can describe aloud what he notices as much or as little as he likes.

- Let your client know there may be times you will repeat back to him his exact words so he can hear them again and notice more about them. If you do the repeating back without having explained this to your client, he is likely to look at you oddly and wonder what is going on, which means his attention will not be on himself.

- Your client's role: You can let your client know that he may surprise himself with some of his answers and that's fine and normal. Expect the unexpected! There are no right or wrong answers, just intuited ones. He should just go with what "comes to mind." In particular when exploring metaphors, I use the phrase *dream logic* to explain why answers can be odd if judged by daily reality standards.

- You may want to explain that you are not going to maintain eye contact (see below) as you would in a normal conversation and that your client doesn't have to either.

- You may want to let your client know that sometimes change occurs spontaneously and at other times it evolves slowly, perhaps over days, weeks, or longer. Letting him know this sows a seed of possibility for change and can relieve the qualms of a client who may be wondering, as the session progresses, if he is "doing it right" or having a "normal" experience.

- If you are conducting a Clean spatial or drawing process, you will want to briefly explain to your client what you and he will be doing, as it is certainly different than a typical talking session. I will save suggestions for the facilitating tips sections of the first spatial and drawing processes as to what you might say; it will make more sense once you have an idea of the processes.

No doubt you will determine for yourself other points you will want to make as you experiment with these techniques. Be sure to take or make opportunities to be a client with these approaches, as it will greatly inform your own facilitating. That and your clients' questions will help you determine what you want to say before you begin a session.

Eye contact

Once you start a Clean process, disengage from normal eye contact with your client. Eye contact just encourages him to converse with you and stay tuned to *your* reactions when what you want him to do is be focused on his *own* reactions. I do not mean to say you will never connect eyes, but, in general, you want to be looking at *the space or place* your questions are referring your client toward rather than at him directly. This could mean looking at a part of his body he has mentioned, at his drawing, at a place in the room, etc.

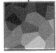

So how will you observe your client's responses, read his body language, and determine his readiness for the next question if you are not looking at him? You will be able to do all that, but wait until he stops expecting your eye contact and starts to get involved in his own process. It usually does not take long. Once he realizes you are not engaging his eyes as we do in most conversations, he will likely stop looking at you. Then you can sneak peeks as needed.

Voice

- Take your time asking questions; do not rush on to the next question. As you slow down, you give the message to your client that it's okay for him to take his time. This will allow him the opportunity to notice details and register feelings. Watch for visual clues, such as turning his head back toward you or seeking eye contact, that suggest he is done responding and processing before asking your next question.

- When asking your questions, pause between phrases or key words in a sentence to create rhythm and emphasis, for example (where dots represent pauses), "And what do you know...from there?"

   I cannot emphasize enough how important it is that you slow down, that you *not* speak at a normal, conversational speed. This enhances your client's mindful inner focus and explorative thinking. Say these Clean questions or directions at a fast clip, and your client will stay in or go right "into his head." That is, he will seek answers from a cognitive place rather than from a place of deeper intuitive knowing. You may be left wondering what the big deal is about Clean processes, when in fact, you have not actually given them their due.

   So practice slowing down…and then slow down even more; I *really* mean speak slowly, putting plenty of pauses between short phrases of a few words, to allow your client plenty of time.

- Subtly convey your curiosity as you ask questions. Your interest, focus, and attention suggest respect for your client, his responses, indeed his very words. This encourages him to get more interested in their details too.

Referring to yourself

In a word: don't! Do not add phrases like "I notice…" "I'm wondering…" "Tell me about…". When you do, you are drawing attention to yourself and suggesting that explaining himself to you is what your client is there for. But it's not about you! Remember: a Clean session is about helping a client get to know himself better, not about helping you understand him better. Referring to yourself takes your client away from his experiencing of himself and suggests he should take you into account.

Taking notes

You may want to take some notes of what your client says, especially if you are using Clean Language questions that require that you repeat your client's exact words back. Certainly you will need some notes for Clean Space, Clean Action, and Clean Action Space. What should you write down?

This is where practice is helpful. You will know you are not writing down enough if you cannot repeat your client's words accurately when needed. You are writing too much if you cannot keep up with what your client is saying or if you find at the end of a session that you have written down much more than you needed to refer to again. Every facilitator will have different needs and wants, so experiment. Get a friend or colleague to practice with before trying a session with a client if you are concerned about looking ill-prepared. For most lean Clean processes, you need to keep track of only what it is the client *wants* and key words, especially metaphors and internal resources, about which we will get into more detail later.

Using charts

There are charts in the back of this book with scripts for each of the processes with the basic questions and in some cases, optional additional questions to use. You might want to make a copy of the one you will be practicing so you can easily hold it as you facilitate without having to juggle this book. You may also want to reduce its size on a copy machine so you can use it without your clients' awareness.

Feel free to change the format of the charts. Everyone has his own best way of learning and organizing information (as will be abundantly clear when you observe a Clean session!). Experiment and find your own best way of supporting your facilitations.

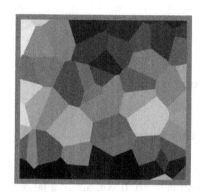

Priming the Pump

If you want to get water from a well that has an old-fashioned pump, the kind with a long handle, you won't get much with your first few pumps. You've got to prime the pump. That is, the pipe has to be filled first with water from its source.

The Clean processes in this first section serve a similar priming purpose. They encourage your client to leave behind his daily world and settle into his session with a different focus. With just a few questions and in just a few minutes, these techniques tap into your client's subconscious, that veritable well of information, and call up its information. Simple as the processes are, they will help you get a flow of information from a deeper, inner place quickly and efficiently.

PROCESS #1: CLEAN SITUATING

Designed to:

> Get you and your client located in right relation to one another
> Connect your client to his intuitive knowing

Useful for: Starting off any session you hold *in person* with your client

Time to allot: It depends on a number of considerations. In a small space and with a client who has done it before, this usually takes a matter of 10 seconds or so. If you are in a large space (for example, if you are an equine therapist in a spacious field), it could take several minutes of wandering around for your client to answer these few questions.

Materials needed: none

The Clean Situating process

Clean Situating is not one of David Grove's titles, though it is a technique he and his co-developer from the 1980s and 1990s, psychotherapist Cei Davies Linn, developed. It seems to be one of the few ideas Grove did not label, so I am left to improvise. Clean Seating does not cover it all, nor does Clean Standing, so I think of it as Clean Situating.

This is about establishing where your client and you will be in the space you are using for your session. There are likely positions for the two of you that best allow your client to focus and open up, to allow new knowledge to emerge. Only your client can know what that is.

You may need to allow a few extra minutes if this is your client's first time with this process. These questions will likely surprise him, and they may take a bit of explaining and experimenting with. Once your client has done this once and experienced the differences in determining where you and he will be, you will need to ask these questions only when first entering your space, and he will usually do it without delay.

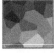

I encourage you not to skip this starting process no matter how many sessions a client has done. What can end up happening is that the client returns to the same place, perhaps out of habit, and that location becomes downloaded with a particular problem, emotion, and/ or chunk of information. Then every time your client sits there, that is what he will tap into. A seat that has been the place where he has explored a problem time and again can become the place where he remains stuck in the problem. Many of the techniques you will learn in this book involve moving around to multiple spaces in part to circumvent this very problem. But whether you are using a movement-oriented, verbal, or drawing/art-making technique, these two simple questions at the start of every session will get you off to a good start. Try it with your next client.

Clean Situating script

Step #1: Establishing his position
As your client enters your session space (this means before he sits down!), ask:

> **"And where would you like to be?"**

Step #2: Establishing the facilitator's position
Once your client selects a space, settles in, and looks at you, ask:

> **"And where would you like me to be?"**

Gesture to several possible alternatives in the room, or if there is only one other chair, make it clear it can be moved by saying so or with gestures.

What is happening?

With this seemingly simple exercise that takes but a minute or so and sometimes mere seconds, a myriad of things happen.

1. You give your client an opportunity to quiet down and focus, to set aside time and space to do some personal work. By doing so in a way that doesn't invite cognitive analysis, assessment, or even much talking at all, you are turning down the volume of that part of the client and turning up the volume of his inner voice.

2. There aren't particularly logical answers to these Clean Situating questions; they don't have wrong or right answers. To answer "And where would you like me to be?" your client has to go to a place of intuitive knowing. When he draws upon his intuitive sense of what seems right, he projects that inner knowing into the space in and around him. Spatial relationships, such as location and distance in front, behind, above, etc., begin to take on meaning. The space begins to become what Grove called *psychoactive*, that is, it fills with information from the client's inner experience, projected outward.

3. You subtly signal to your client that this is *his* session. You may be the expert he has come to, but he is the ultimate expert on himself. You are expecting and respecting his input, right from the get-go. Just as he takes on some responsibility for the setup, so he must take some of the responsibility for determining and acting upon what he will learn for himself.

Clean Language is about subtlety and exactness.

Notice you don't ask, "And where would you like to *sit* or *stand*?" but "And where would you like to *be*?" This gives your client the maximum flexibility to consult his inner sense of the right place and position for him at that moment. I have had clients choose to lie on a massage table; sit on the floor; and stand, looking out a window. Who knows what information their positions' perspective lends them?

Be careful not to add anything to the question either. Think of it as a ritual phrase, if you will, where you use the exact same wording every time. It's awfully easy to get chatty and thoughtlessly add words like "And where would you be *most comfortable*?" How un-Clean! This directs your client to select a place with a particular feeling, purpose, and/or priority of your choosing.

Don't rush your client.

Just because he has stopped walking or even sat down doesn't mean your client is finished feeling out the space, scanning his body, and seeing whether this setup feels intuitively right. Look at his body language to let you know he is ready for your next question. Usually a client will let out his breath, sit back, settle his shoulders, and/or look at you directly when he is ready to move on.

FAQs Frequently Asked Questions

I have a small office. How can I give my client a choice?

To whatever degree possible, invite your client to arrange himself and you in the space. Even a small shift in position or angle can make a difference. Be careful not to "claim" a particular chair by, for example, standing next to it with your hand on its back while you ask your client where he would like to be. Ideally, the available chairs will be relatively similar; if you have a big padded office chair and a smaller, typical side chair, it sends a message that the latter is yours. You are not really giving an open invitation! Stand clear, avoid suggesting any particular place with your eyes, and truly let the client choose. If he chooses the chair in which you usually sit, be flexible and go with it. With the sorts of Clean questions you will be asking, all kinds of interesting things could happen!

What if I ask, "And where would you like to be?" and my client says, "Oh, anywhere is fine. Where do you usually sit?"

In the friendliest of ways, try not to settle for this answer. It is not unusual for the first-time client to think choosing his place is unimportant. Or he may want to please you, or perhaps he is worried there is a wrong answer. Or he may not be used to tapping into his own preferences. There are numerous reasons a client might deflect this question. But your client's self-exploration starts right here, in this moment, with these two simple Clean Situating questions. Think through now how you will reply.

If a client of mine gives this kind of response, I usually say something like "Feel free to experiment. See if you have a preference! Try several places." Once he settles I will ask where he wants me to be. If he says, "Anywhere," I might be playful to establish a friendly atmosphere: maybe I will go to the far side of the room, or turn my back, or stand behind my client. My client usually chuckles and suggests a chair. Once I am seated, I will ask, "How is this?" and I will move my chair around a bit to make it clear I can easily adjust it and to give my client a chance to experience how even a small change can feel different. I may change angles, face directly toward my client or turn perpendicular. My client begins to notice it *does* make a difference, and he will direct me. You can invite your client once again to make similar adjustments.

Some clients like to look out a window. And I deliberately keep at least one wall in my office free of any decorations so my clients can choose to face a "blank page" with no distractions.

If your client moves himself or you, be sure to check in again until he has approved *both* his position and yours without having changed either by asking something like "And is this okay now?"

For the first-time client, I add "Feel free to ask me to move or move yourself during the session if it seems right to do so."

What if my client suggests something uncomfortable or impractical?

Feel free to use your common sense. If your client suggests that you take a position that is truly uncomfortable, unsafe, or for some other reason just will not work well, redirect. You can still stay *clean*.

Explain your standards simply and briefly: "I don't hear well out of this ear" or "That fence is electrified" (as it might be for an equine therapy session).

And then ask, as needed: "And where is another space you would like to be/you would like me to be?"

But whenever you can, make adjustments to meet your client's needs. You want to honor his tuning into himself for information. Learning to again hear one's inner voice is a great gift to someone who has lost that ability, and it can start with Clean Situating.

PROCESS #2: CLEAN START

Designed to:
> Get your client and his representation of his topic of inquiry located in right relation to one another
> Connect your client to his intuitive knowing

Useful for:
> Starting off many Clean spatial sessions
> Helping a client who is only vaguely aware of what he wants to address
> Quieting the "on-the-go," the "in-his-head," or the "can't-stop-talking-for-a-moment" client
> Getting a symbolic representation for an issue a client described in cognitive terms

Time to allot: usually 3–6 minutes

Materials needed:
> Paper, writing/drawing utensil(s)
> Optional: a selection of objects

The Clean Start process

This is another quick technique you can use to begin a session. Your client begins by writing or sketching his topic of inquiry on a piece of paper. I find post-its and markers work well. If you choose to use them, you may want to have several colors of both paper and markers on hand to give your client options. Who knows what meaning he will make of the colors he picks, meanings that you may or may not hear about, that may be conscious or subconscious?

Rather than having the client write or draw words, another option is to offer a variety of objects or invite the client to bring an object to represent his issue or topic of inquiry. Grove called them *co-inspiring objects*. Like all client-selected metaphors, they hold unique meaning for the client, and attributes of the object contribute to the client's emerging understanding. The client always chooses the object. Stay Clean; don't make suggestions!

As the client places his paper or object somewhere to see what he can discover, the Clean Start process slows him down. As he locates the paper/object and himself in what seem like the right positions, he begins to *psychoactivate* the space with his inner knowing.

Clean Start script

Step #1: Establishing the client's want or topic of inquiry [x]

Give *one or both* of these clean directives:

> **"And draw or write what you would like to have happen…or know more about."**
> (gesturing to the paper and markers)

or

> **"And choose an object to represent what would you like to have happen…or to know more about."** (gesturing to your collection of objects or around the space)

Normally when we speak conversationally, we do not insert the word *have* before *happen*, as we do in this question. David Grove experimented to determine just what words he would use, and I have come to deeply appreciate the value of this extra little word for setting the question apart as an invitation for a special sort of exploration. There is a rhythm to it that invites a different sort of processing. So be sure you are saying this phrase exactly as written!

I have noticed facilitators often add the word "today" to their question. Decide with care if you want to ask "And what would you like to have happen today?"; it does, potentially, make for an entirely different question. In general, I recommend you start by leaving it off and seeing where your client's attention is focused. You can always ask the question again later, adding the word "today" to bring some kind of focus or closure to the session if you feel it is needed.

Step #2: Setting up

You will refer to your client's topic as "that" from now on as you gesture toward the paper/object, pausing to allow your client the mental time to fill in the blank.

> **"And place that** (gesturing to the paper/object) **where it seems…right."** (gesturing around the space)

Be sure to keep yourself out of any space your client seems to be considering. You don't want to be in his psycho-activated space. Step back behind and to the side of him if you are standing. Move your chair out of the client's line of sight if he seems to be locating a spot close to you.

Once your client has placed the paper/object, direct:

> **"And place yourself where you are in relation to that** (gesture to the paper/object)**…now."**

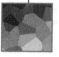

Sometimes this directive confuses the first-time client, as there can be a bit of a learning curve to getting the hang of sensing a space that conveys information. I generally find that if you gesture again to the paper or object, pause…and repeat the directive as you look around the space (making a sweeping gesture) and your client figures it out. If your client is still stymied, try inviting him to "Take all the time you need to walk about and find the space where you are in relation to that (gesture toward the paper again)…now."

Step #3: Aligning the spaces

Clean Start is primarily about giving your client opportunities to reconsider his placement of his paper/object and himself and to further refine them according to distance, angle, height, direction, and position. *It is not necessary to ask every question listed below, nor is this the required order in which to ask them.* These questions are set off in pairs only for the purpose of making them easier to read. And remember: you do *not* have to ask them in pairs.

> **"And are you in the right space?"**
> **"And is [x] in the right space?"**
>
> **"And are you at the right height?"**
> **"And is [x] at the right height?"**
>
> **"And are you facing the right direction?"**
> **"And is [x] facing the right direction?"**
>
> **"And are you at the right angle?"**
> **"And is [x] at the right angle?"**
>
> **"And are you at the right distance from [x]?"**
> **"And is [x] the right distance from you?"**
>
> **"And are you in the right position?"**
> **"And is [x] in the right position?"**

After much experimentation, David Grove felt six to be the minimum number of questions needed to prompt emergence. So you could aim for six questions, but you will undoubtedly respond to your client.

- If your client does a lot of moving about and rearranging with each of your questions, you may want to ask more than six questions, even coming back to some of them until the paper/object and your client seem to be settled in and you are getting a lot of "*Yes, it's right*" answers. Who knows what is going on inside the client, but it would appear this process is a helpful invitation to sort some things out or make them more accessible that may not even be at a level of conscious awareness yet.

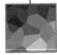

- If your client has done this before, you may notice he is doing adjustments on his own without your asking the questions. That's fine; you may decide you do not need to do a full six questions before moving on to the next step.

Step #4: Synthesizing

Once your client confirms that all is situated correctly, ask:

> **"And what do you know…from there?"**

Optional to ask one time (remember: you are just panning for gold here):

> **"And is there anything else you know…from there?"**

What is happening?

As your client takes a few moments to go through the Clean Start process, all kinds of things start happening. If these sound familiar, it is because they are the same sorts of things that happen with Clean Situating, but this time the relationship being established is between your client and his inner content rather than with you.

1. You are quieting down and focusing your client, encouraging him to set aside time and space to do some personal work. By doing so in a way that doesn't invite cognitive analysis, assessment, or even much talking at all, you are encouraging him to turn down the volume of those parts and turn up the volume of his inner voice.

2. You are encouraging your client to establish a *psychoactive* space. When he draws upon his intuitive sense of what seems right, he projects that inner knowing into the space inside and around him. Spatial relationships, such as location and distance in front, behind, above, etc., begin to take on meaning.

3. You are subtly signaling to the client that this is *his* session. He is the expert on himself, and he has the primary responsibility for it, right from the get-go. He determines the topic of inquiry, and all the information you help him gather will come from him alone.

4. By asking the client to note where it seems right for him and the paper/object to be, you introduce the idea that these locations could be different. You set the stage for exploring different perspectives, as either the paper/object or the client could move.

Example: Jaime

Jaime is a college senior who doesn't know what she wants to do after graduating. Offering her a selection of color post-its and markers to choose from, I invite Jaime to select a marker and pad. She chooses a yellow pad and a blue marker.

Facilitator: **And write or draw what you would like to have happen…or to know more about.**

Jaime sums up her dilemma in one word, which she puts on a post-it: *career*.

Facilitator: **And place that** (gesturing from the paper to the rest of the space) **where it seems…right.**

Jaime places her post-it on a blank wall at eye level between two windows.

Facilitator: **And place yourself where you are in relation to** career (gesturing to the post-it)… **now.**

Step #3: Aligning the spaces

I wait until Jaime has selected a spot, looks toward the post-it, appears settled, and looks back expectantly.

Facilitator: **And is** career (gesturing to the paper) **at the right height?**

She considers the post-it and nods.

Facilitator: **And are you at the right distance?**

Jaime takes two steps back and then returns to where she had been and nods.

Facilitator: **And are you at the right angle?**

She takes a few steps to the right, rotates to face the paper, and stops.

Jaime: *Okay.*

Facilitator: **And is** career (gesturing to the paper) **at the right angle?**

Jamie adjusts the paper, returns to her space, and looks up at me, waiting for the next question.

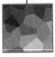

Facilitator:	**And are you facing the right direction?**
Jaime:	*Yes.*
Facilitator:	**And are you at the right height?**
Jaime:	*Yes. Yes, this is right.*

Step #4: Synthesizing

Facilitator:	**And what do you know…from there?**
Jaime:	*I'm graduating from college in a few months. I want to explore what I might do. I'm an art major. I love to paint, to be creative, to work with others on team projects. But I don't know how to translate those passions into a job!*
Facilitator:	**And is there anything else you know…from there?**
Jaime:	*I don't know anything about a career. I'm sort of at a loss.*

An "I don't know" answer does not mean you have done anything wrong or that Clean Start has failed somehow. We will pick up Jaime's session with another Clean process later in the book to demonstrate where you might go from here.

 FAQs *Frequently Asked Questions*

What size paper works best?

The answer will be different depending on the person. If you are going to be facilitating one of the techniques involving drawing, I usually offer copy paper, letter or legal size. Sometimes it is great to have a larger piece like flip chart paper or even a butcher's roll of paper available.

Then there are times it is good to use post-it notes. For techniques that use space, I find it advantageous to give my client a small piece of paper that encourages him to be concise, as his focus will be on the space rather than on the written word or drawing.

And you might want some masking tape in case your client wants to put the paper on the wall. (I find the post-its start to fall off after awhile without extra tape, which can get most distracting!) If you are working outside, be sure to have some weights for the post-its so they don't blow around.

When do I suggest writing/drawing on a piece of paper versus using an object?

Why not offer both options? The more control for the session you give the client, the better. If you cannot keep a collection of objects (perhaps you are not working in your office or are outside), suggest ahead of time that the client bring an object, find one in whatever space you are in, or stick to paper.

You are going to be learning some Clean techniques that work with moving about in space and some that work with the written word or drawings. Both the paper and object lend themselves to being moved about in space, so either is fine if you expect to move on to a Clean technique using space.

If you are going to work with the written word or drawing, then presumably you will want to start with the paper option. If you are working with young children, you might sense that an object or drawing would work better than the written word.

Some clients may be overwhelmed by a blank page; using an object might be helpful for such a client. Generally, I would say use your common sense and consider your individual client. And again, experiment! You might be surprised by what happens when you try something new.

What kind of objects should I have available?

There is no "should" here. Offer a variety. I encourage you to have some natural objects as well as manmade ones. A feather, a rock, a shell. An old-fashioned pen. A dog tag, a key, a padlock. A coin, a button, a decorative star. Look around the house. What seems to invite multiple interpretations and associations?

Avoid having so many objects that your client gets caught up in looking over your "museum collection." Let your client know that if none of the objects seem right, he can always choose to write or draw an object on paper. Sometimes a client might have something in her purse, his wallet, or book bag that will seem right.

PROCESS #3: CLEAN LANGUAGE AND THE BEFORE OUR SESSION SHEET

BEFORE OUR SESSION

To have a focus to begin our session, please answer the following question. Free free to write as much or as little as you like.

What would you like to have happen?

Draw a sketch of what this would look like. NO artistic talent is required; stick figures are fine. Use another piece of paper or the back of this one if you need more room.

Designed to:

    Get your client to focus on an intention for the session

    Get your client's metaphor(s) for what he wants

    Clarify any issue

    Help your client learn more about his resource metaphor(s)

Useful for:

    Starting a session

    Getting metaphors from a verbal into a physical form

Time to allot: 5–8 minutes, though some clients report spending much longer. Your client can bring this sheet with him, already completed.

Materials needed:

    Email version of sheet to be filled out ahead of time

    or

    Paper for drawing (Copy paper, letter or business size, is easy to purchase, store, and carry around. At times, you may prefer to offer a larger size like flip chart paper or a butcher roll.)

    Markers

    Firm drawing surface

    Before Our Session sheet

The Before Our Session sheet

The concept for the Before Our Session sheet I provide a client in advance of his session comes from James Lawley and Penny Tompkins. I have experimented with variations over the years, adding a question, deleting another. Experiment to find one that is right for you and your context; just be sure to keep it short, simple, and Clean.

I email my client this sheet and ask him to bring this sheet to our session or fax/email it to me earlier in the day. I encourage him *not* to do this well in advance of the session; that way, the issue he selects is more likely to feel relevant that day. The process of preparing the sheet means he will have spent time thinking about what he wants to address in the session. It seems to get us down to business more efficiently. It is also a fine way to convey the message that your client is in control of the content he will work with in the session.

I begin a session by inviting my client to read or describe what he has written and drawn. This gets him connected with his issue in a mindful way again and gives me his exact words to refer to. You will find that sometimes clients will read aloud the words they have written with no changes. Other times, they will add or change words. It is all part of their self-discovery process.

Clean Language questions

I am going to start you off with two basic CLQs you can ask your client in addition to the one on the top of the sheet (**"What would you like to have happen?"**). You can ask these next questions about the exact words your client writes on the top section of the page or verbally adds to that description. You can also ask him about the words he uses to describe his drawings.

When [x] is a word or short phrase the client uses, start by repeating what your client says, followed by one of these CLQs:

> **"And** [client's word(s)]."
> **"And what kind of** [x] **is that** [x]**?"**

> **"And** [client's word(s)]."
> **"And is there anything else about that** [x]**?"**

Example: Diane

Drawing: A simple stick figure, facing out with feet spread slightly wide apart, holding a stick.

Diane: *I have a coworker that, frankly, bullies me. I've tried avoiding her, but that's not always possible. I want to be better at coping with confrontation.*

Facilitator: **And** you want to be better at coping with confrontation. **And what kind of** coping **is that** coping**?**

Diane: *Coping means I stay strong even when I'm confronted.*

Facilitator: **And** stay strong. **And is there anything else about that** stay strong**?**

Diane: *It's like holding up to a strong wind and not being blown over or even off course.*

Facilitator: **And** holding up to a strong wind. **And is there anything else about** holding up to a strong wind**?**

Diane: *Even though there's wind, I stand up to it. And I have a stick to help me.*

Facilitator: **And** a stick to help you. **And what kind of** stick is that stick**?**

Diane: *Actually, it's a walking stick. Huh! When I drew it, I thought it might be a cane or something to fight somebody off with; but no, it's a walking stick. Huh!*

Sometimes your client will be surprised; then you know he has learned something about himself or what he needs that he did not consciously know before. And that is what I am looking to have happen. As a facilitator of my client's exploration, I am not trying to fix anything, not trying to problem solve for him. I am simply extending and deepening his attention on what is coming up for him, encouraging him to notice more about it with simple, Clean questions.

The magnetic pull of problems

It is generally assumed in our culture that the way to approach problems is to analyze them, to *problem solve*. Problems draw us like magnets! Your interest and concern about your client's life may tempt you to ask questions about the what's and why's of his past or current problems. But insight into the historical sources of and reasons for problems isn't necessarily all that helpful, and it may not be the best use of your limited time together. Filling you in on what he already knows is time you are not spending helping your client move from where he is to where he wants to be.

In the example above, notice that I did not ask about the client about her coworker or the bullying. That is because it would likely lead to a lengthy telling of the stories of past issues, stories she already knows and I do not need to know. Probably her focus would go toward the coworker, about whom we can do little to change. Likely the client will feel frustrated and discouraged as she goes through her complaints.

What to ask about instead

Instead of getting mired in the story of this particular office problem, this Clean process can help Diane clarify how she would like to respond instead. It helps her get clearer on what she wants and helps her discover her metaphors for the *internal resources* she needs to accomplish that.

What words/phrases do you ask about with these Clean Language questions?

1. Words/phrases that describe what the client would *like*

2. Metaphors

3. Resources

If you are unclear yet as to what I mean, this book is full of examples of each of these in the client session transcripts. Let me take a moment here, however, to talk about resources in particular.

Resources

Resources are those things that the client identifies as helpful. They could be people, objects, skills, knowledge, or creative ideas, for example. Clean processes are particularly conducive to helping clients become more aware of internal resources they often overlook: their supportive feelings such as competence, confidence, and focus.

Just what constitutes a resource depends on the client and the situation. In one context, being relaxed is a beneficial or resourceful state. In another context, being energized and excited is, whereas being laid back would be a problem. So be listening to the whole of what your client is saying to determine what acts as a resource *for him* in the context he is describing.

Diane said she needs a particular kind of coping. I am going to trust her wisdom that that is just the resourceful state she needs information about right now. I zoom in her attention on the details to find out more about what better coping is like for her. (I would keep going in the example above, finding out about the resourceful stick.) If that does not resolve her problem, she will at least approach her situation with a new perspective, supported by better developed resources.

This lean approach is not sufficient in every instance. At times, a client will not be able to articulate what he wants. He is simply not there yet. Or awareness alone is not enough. To handle this situation and for more extensive work with resources and metaphors using Clean Language, I again refer you to my two workbooks on Clean Language and Symbolic Modeling (Campbell, 2012, 2013).

FAQs | *Frequently Asked Questions*

What if my client doesn't just say a sentence, but a whole paragraph? Do I repeat it all?

In a word, no. Select a word/short phrase that relates to (1) a metaphor (2) a resource or (3) concerns what the client wants. Repeat it to acknowledge it and to single it out for your client's attention. Then ask the Clean question about that word/short phrase.

Can I ask about a longer phrase?

Be sure you break it down into smaller chunks and ask several questions. If you ask about a lot at once, you are liable to get a cognitive answer because there are so many pieces for your client to process. Ask about only a word or two, and suddenly the client can answer more intuitively. He may, for example, notice something about his word choice that surprises and informs him, especially if it is about a metaphor.

Can I ask about more than one part of the client's paragraph?

Yes, indeed. This is why you might want to take a few notes. But remember, you are just "priming the pump" with the limited amount of Clean Language you have learned thus far. You may not get to questions about everything that could be significant.

As a general rule of thumb for beginners, if you have a verbose client and are at a loss as to where to start, I suggest you ask about things *in the drawing* as opposed to other things the client talks about. It's there in front of you to help you remember it. And as it is among the few things the client chose to depict from all he verbally says, likely something about it is significant.

Also pay careful attention to the times when your client appears to be thinking or processing something, and give him uninterrupted time to do that. He may take the opportunity to talk about what seems important to him that you have not asked about. Don't rush him.

Once you have some experience with working with the Before our Session sheet, you will no doubt get clearer on which words/phrases you will likely choose.

How long should I spend asking questions about what's on the sheet?

It will depend on what your client says and what else you have in mind for the session. Your client's answers may offer an opportunistic time to segue into another Clean process, or you may have another professional modality to apply.

Remember though, you are *panning* for gold: ask only a question or two about any one detail and then move on to another. Let the higher level awareness *emerge* from the cluster of small bits of information. Be prepared to find that all the bits needed may not come out with the Before Our Session sheet; it is just the start.

What if my client starts describing what's on the page and wants to change it?

That's fine. In fact, I let my client know before we start looking at his sheet that he is free to add or in any way change what he has brought. After all, the completed sheet is not a goal in and of itself; it is simply a tool for enhancing the client's awareness of himself and what he wants.

Sometimes clients write just a sentence; other times, they fill the page. Sometimes they do the drawings, sometimes not. Your job is to work with whatever the client brings.

Caution: If a client changes something on his page, do not ask in effect "Why did you make that change?" Notice that *no Clean question ever uses the word "why."* To answer why, your client may go to a more cognitive, analytical place to find the answer, which is not what we are going for with Clean; we are seeking a deeper mind/body wisdom. If he does not have an answer, he may start to be distracted by the thought that he should. Or he may feel he has to justify himself; he might get defensive. None of these is a direction you want to send your client's attention in.

What you want is to keep his attention on his own words or image, right where his awareness and knowing is now…and then use a Clean question to take it just a step at a time further.

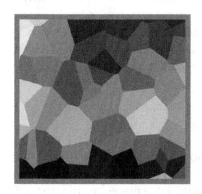

When Space Becomes Psychoactive

CLEAN SPATIAL PROCESSES

It seems altogether too simple, really. You select a topic you want to explore: perhaps you want to know more about how you might handle a relationship issue or what steps you need to take to share your passion with a larger audience. With just a few guiding questions from your facilitator, something extraordinary starts happening.

You discover information about a topic or issue when you stand in one spot in a room, and when you walk to another spot, you find something additional or even contradictory. What sort of magic trick is this, you may wonder? How is it I can sense this so clearly, so physically? How is it that I have an emotional response to this too? I really do feel excited or confused or energized or clear for the first time. It seems impossible, and yet it happens easily!

David Grove developed several Clean processes that invite clients to project their inner experiences into the space around them. When space holds information from the client's mind/body system with which he actively engages, Grove termed it *psychoactive*.

Like puzzle pieces

If you have ever put together a jigsaw puzzle, you know how hard it would be to find the pieces you need if they stay piled in a heap. But get a surface to spread the pieces out on, one big enough so you can see them all, and there they are: the edge pieces...or the parts of the cat's eye...or those bits of sky. You may not have been searching for something specific, particularly at the start. You may have only a vague idea of what might be useful—until you find it.

Clean spatial processes allow your client to take what is jumbled inside and lay it out before him. Sometimes he is clear on what he needs to know more about; sometimes he has only a general idea. As he journeys around, visiting spaces he chooses, relevant pieces of his puzzle reveal themselves.

By helping your client spread his inner information out around him, these Clean processes help him grasp a sense of the *whole*. With this broad vision, he is better able to understand the relationship between the individual parts, whether they are parts of himself or parts of a problem or project. From this perspective, he can identify priorities, imagine new possibilities, and set intentions that best serve the whole of him.

Remember the description of emergence science in Section 1? Clean spatial processes are Grovian ways of creating the conditions needed to amass multiple bits of information. Holding them in time and space allows an emergent new order of structure and understanding to manifest.

Notice I use the word *allows*. As the facilitator, you are creating the *conditions* for change; you cannot force it. And you should not blame yourself if it does not occur. Change occurs if and when the client's system needs it and is ready for it.

Uses

The processes in this section that move a client around to various spaces are all useful for helping him:

- Consider multiple options
- Sort out complex issues
- Consider something from new or multiple perspectives

Precisely because moving about in space is such an unusual way to access information for most people, these techniques can be very valuable for clients who tend to live in their heads and can suffer from "analysis paralysis."

For clients who are naturally kinesthetic in their orientation, these techniques can be great favorites. They help these clients tap into information they may feel they can't find other ways, yet feel so "right." Moving helps them think, and with these processes, they can finally "hear themselves."

But these processes are not just for special cases. All clients can potentially find these Clean experiences help them access unexpected "gold." Approaching an issue, literally, from different physical perspectives can be transformational.

FACILITATING TIPS

We will be covering three lean Clean spatial processes in this section that use psycho-activated space as their medium: Clean Spinning, Clean Networks, and Clean Space. But before we do, let me go over some suggestions for how to best facilitate these experiences for your client.

Preparing your client

How you set up your contract with your client as to what he wants and can expect from the session will vary depending on your profession. I expect you already have a model worked out for that. In terms of the Clean spatial processes, your role as facilitator is to provide some structure for your client's exploration. You give short directives and ask simple questions, sticking pretty closely to a script with little variation. In addition to the suggestions on page 20 (the Preparing your client section), here is an idea of the sorts of things you might want to say to your client in preparation for the spatial processes in this section.

> "[Name of Clean process] is an active way of exploring a topic or goal you have. It's quite simple, really. I'm going to be doing two things: asking you to find spaces and then asking you "What do you know from there?" and possibly a few other similarly simple questions. This will give you a chance to collect the information that you are already aware of and very likely to discover there is more you know about your topic or goal than you realized.

"My role is basically to give you some structure and keep you exploring. You don't even have to tell me the actual content that you are exploring. You can answer the questions aloud or simply to yourself. This is about *self-exploration*, not *self-explanation*. You may notice a shift or change immediately, or it could evolve gradually after you leave here.

"The session will probably take about _____ minutes, and then we'll have some time to talk about what you discovered and what you would like to have happen if you're open to that. Any questions before we begin?"

Spend some time preparing an explanation for your client ahead of time. Without one, you may find your client baulks at what seem like unusual questions or repeatedly interrupts his process to clarify what he is meant to do.

Your tone and demeanor

Keep your voice neutral and accepting. You want to avoid sounding conversational to discourage your client from trying to engage you in his process. Keeping your voice rhythmically and tonally consistent encourages your client to enter into and stay in his psychoactive space.

Eye contact

Avoid a lot of eye contact with the client. Aim to keep your eyes on the *spaces*, directing your energy and attention (and thus guiding your client's) toward them rather than on the connection between the two of you.

Where to position yourself

You are no doubt familiar with the concept of personal space. You know when someone stands too close to you; it feels like they are "in your space." It can be very uncomfortable and distracts you from what you are concentrating on. In these Clean sessions, be careful not to step into a client's space or walk across the area between his spaces. This can be distracting at best, invasive at worst. Make an exaggerated point of giving the spaces your client chooses wide berth; it will convey to your client a deep sense of respect. This means that as more spaces are added and the space between them expands, you may need to move to stay outside the perimeter of the psycho-active spaces. This will make more sense as you read on.

We will be covering three Clean spatial processes, starting with the shortest and simplest to help you easily master these new ways of facilitating.

PROCESS #4: CLEAN SPINNING

Designed to:

Help your client quickly discover information from multiple perspectives

Enhance clarity

Get your client in touch with his intuitive knowing

Useful for:

A quick start—another way to prime the pump

Inserting into another Clean process at an appropriate moment

Time to allot: 5–10 minutes

Materials needed: none

The Clean Spinning process

It is extraordinary how the subconscious will take opportunities to make meaning of simple objects, actions, movements, events, etc. I have known clients to find meaning in a passing plane, the patterns in a rug, a cloud passing in front of the sun, a phone ringing. You name it! My clients never stop surprising me, and I never get bored in a Clean session. The surprising things clients discover with this technique are great examples.

Clean Spinning could not be simpler. You are simply inviting your client to turn around repeatedly and notice what he discovers. As your client spins around, he is altering his perspective of the space around him, literally, and in turn (no pun intended!), his inner world. You will notice this process begins like Clean Start.

The Clean Spinning script

Step #1: Establishing the client's want or topic of inquiry

Give *one or both* of these clean directives:

> **"And draw or write what you would like to have happen…or know more about."**
> (gesturing to the paper and markers)

> or

> **"And choose an object to represent what would you like to have happen…or to know more about."** (gesturing to your collection of objects or around the space)

Step #2: Setting up

When your client has articulated his answer enough to describe it in a word or short phrase, what we will call [x], direct him by saying:

> **"And place that** (gesturing to the paper or object) **where it seems…right."**

> **"And place yourself where you are in relation to that** (gesturing to the paper or object)**…now."**

Step #3: Gathering information

> **"And what do you know…from there?"**

Once your client has responded, you are going to have him rotate in that space. Direct:

> **"And turn in either direction…until it seems right to stop."**

When he has stopped turning and seems settled in (perhaps turning his head to look at you), ask:

> **"And what do you know…from there?"**

Repeat Steps #3 to #5 more times, asking:

> **"And turn again…until it seems right to stop."**

> **"And what do you know…from there?"**

Step #4: Synthesizing

As your client turns and faces his topic (written, drawn, or an object), ask:

> **"And what do you know…now?"**

> **"And what difference…does knowing that…make?"**

Thus, your client will have identified four to six spaces. Grove's ideal was six, but I find clients often turn in a circle, making quarter turns, ending where they began. This often has a feeling of completeness about it, and I don't press for more spaces.

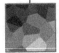

Options

1. You can occasionally ask, particularly if the client's answer is short or the direction is what Grove called a "sweet spot," one that seems to hold significant information:

   "And is there anything else you know...from there?"

   or at the end:

   "And is there anything else you know...now?"

2. You can add a Clean Language question if, for example, your client seems to be wanting to stay in a space (for example, his eyes might be closed, and he seems to be concentrating hard). Or if he mentions a metaphor, help him get a bit more detail.

   Example CLQs:

   "And what kind of [y] is that [y]?" (about a word(s) the client has said)

   "And is there anything else about that [y]?"

   But do not ask more than one or two CLQs at any one space, and do not ask them at every turn. You are only panning the surface for gold, not digging deeply. It is important to keep your client *moving*.

   And that is Clean Spinning. Couldn't be simpler. But don't be surprised if your client discovers something profound. It may not even sound profound to you, but he will have *experienced* an insight, not just thought of it, and that can make a huge difference.

Example: Luis

Facilitator: **And draw or write what you would like to have happen...or know more about.** (gesturing to the paper and markers)

Luis takes a post-it and writes *my management style*. He says aloud:

Luis: *I want to be more aware of my management style.*

Facilitator: **And place that** (gesturing to the paper) **where it seems...right.**

Luis stands, places the paper on the wall, tweaks it a bit, and looks back at the facilitator.

Facilitator: **And place yourself where you are in relation to that** (gesturing to the paper)**...now.**

Luis stands in front of the paper, his knees up against the back of his chair. Dissatisfied, he pushes the chair to the side and backs up a foot. Seemingly satisfied, he looks back at me.

Facilitator: **And what do you know…from there?**

Luis: *I know that what I'm looking at seems cloaked in mist. I really don't know what my style is. I know what I've been taught it should be, but I can't see it clearly.*

Facilitator: **And turn in either direction…until it seems right to stop.**

Luis turns to his right, facing the office door.

Facilitator: **And what do you know…from there?**

Luis: I know I'm aware of my title and posture from the moment I walk in the door at work. I imagine other people seeing me and want to send the right message.

Facilitator: **And** send the right message. **And what kind of** message **is that** right message?

Luis: *That I'm the one to look to. "The buck stops here."*

I have asked one follow-up CLQ, enough for "panning." Despite the fact that he has come up with a metaphor, I decide to move Luis on to the next space. He will carry on with the metaphor or he won't.

Facilitator: **And turn again…until it seems right to stop.**

Luis turns a quarter turn, looking out the window.

Facilitator: **And what do you know…from there?**

Luis: *I know that I tend to focus just on what's in the room. I'm not taking a long-distance view, a long-term view.*

Again I make no comment. I wait patiently while Luis seems to consider his answer. When Luis seems to break away from his thoughts and looks back at me, I continue.

Facilitator: **And turn again…until it seems right to stop.**

Luis turns a quarter turn toward a corner of the room.

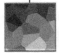

Facilitator: **And what do you know…from there?**

Luis: *For some reason, I'm remembering my father. He was in the military. It was his way or the highway, if you know what I mean. I never bucked his authority, but at times his rigidity made me furious. It was a real relief to go to college.*

Facilitator: **And is there anything else you know…from there?**

Luis: *I suspect I have people under me who want to buck my authority, and I'm not giving them a chance to speak up. Just because the buck stops with me doesn't mean I can't listen.*

Since I trust by now you are getting the hang of Clean Spinning, I am going to skip what might be several more turns in an actual session and complete this example with the final turn and assessment stage.

Facilitator: **And turn again…until it seems right to stop.**

Luis turns to face his post-it, "my management style." Here is the cue that this is the last turn; he is ready to assess what he has learned. I could push on with more turns but decide to end with this space this time.

Facilitator: **And what do you know from there…now?**

Luis: *I see that I'm more like my father than I realized. And I know I want to be more flexible than he was.*

Facilitator: **And what difference…does knowing that…make?**

Luis: *I realize there's space to listen to other's ideas and using them doesn't mean I'm not in charge. I can take a long-term view and that perspective is something I contribute. I've been too focused on the corner and the door.*

At this point, I could use another therapeutic or coaching approach or segue into another Clean process, such as the next one we will cover, Clean Networks. What I do not do is ask for details about what Luis's father was like, what it was like at home before he left for college, or exactly why he thinks he is like his father. I do not get into the history of Luis's story. I simply let Luis find what he finds, what his system is ready for. I am panning for gold and staying Clean.

PROCESS #5: CLEAN NETWORKS

Designed to:
   Clarify any issue or topic
   Open a client to new perspectives and possibilities

Useful for:
   Assessments
   Planning
   Considering the whole of a complex situation
   Sorting out complex feelings
   Self-exploration
   Exploring new possibilities

Time to allot: about 20–40 minutes

Materials needed:
   Post-its, writing instrument, space to move about
   Optional: selection of objects or one the client brings in

The Clean Networks process

In a nutshell, what happens in a Clean Networks session is that your client selects a topic he wants to explore. You invite him to move about the room, selecting spaces that "hold" information and discovering what emerges. One stop at each space is all, with a final return to the first space to take stock of what he has learned. Yes, it is that simple, and yet the results will likely surprise both you and your client.

What do you do besides ask the scripted questions?

Your role is to:

- "Hold the space" for the client's exploration
- Be attentive and accepting
- Speak as little as possible and stay out of the space he is exploring
- Keep in mind the client's original goal

The spaces work with you by:

- Containing information
- Energetically conveying the visceral sense/experience connected with the information
- Allowing the landscape to be experienced as a whole

Clean Networks is one of David Grove's Emergent Knowledge processes. The client collects multiple bits of related information. The facilitator's role is peripheral; he is there as a witness, there to keep the client moving, there to hold the space. As the complexity of the components and their associations increases, the client's mind/body system is challenged to maintain a sense of the whole. If needed, a new structure of organization may emerge naturally.

Clean Networks script

Step #1: Establishing the client's want or topic of inquiry

Give *one or both* of these clean directives:

> **"And draw or write what you would like to have happen...or to know more about."** (gesturing to the paper and markers)

or

> **"And choose an object to represent what would you like to have happen...or to know more about."** (gesturing to your collection of objects or around the space)

Step #2: Setting Up

Once the client's answer is on paper or he has selected an object, direct:

> **"And place that** (gesturing to the paper) **where it seems...right."**

> **"And place yourself where you are in relation to that** (gesturing to the paper or object)**...now."**

Step #3: Gathering Information

> **"And what do you know...from there?"**

Facilitate your client to find additional spaces and what information each holds.
Direct:

> **"And find another space."**

Let your client settle into a space. He will usually look at you directly or say okay or in some other way signal he is done. Then ask:

> **"And what do you know...from there?"**

Repeat this pair of questions until your client has identified and explored about five or six spaces. We discussed already that David Grove believed six spaces create a special synergy for knowledge to emerge. You can experiment with this yourself. You may find you vary the number based on the client and/or on what comes up in any particular session.

Usually the first couple of spaces reveal information that the client already seems familiar with; there is little new here. Typically around the fourth space, things get more interesting. What emerges is either new information or a new level of awareness of an issue. Keep going! Your steadying presence holds the space and encourages your client to push through confusion or frustration to uncover still more new information. Your calm, neutral tone implies that this is normal. After all, if what your client was after was only what he already knew, he would have little reason to come to you in the first place.

Step #4: Synthesizing

Once you have established and explored about six spaces, have your client go back to his first space by directing:

"And return to your first space." (gesturing toward the space)

He has now returned to the space that held what knowing he had when he began the session. Let him settle in. Then ask:

"And what do you know from there…now?"

"And what difference…does knowing that…make?"

The Clean Networks session ends here. Invite your client to pick up his own post-its; they're likely to have emotional resonance for him. Whether he keeps them or throws them away, let it be his choice. If you touch them, it could feel like you are "stepping on" his space.

Options

You can add one of these CLQs at any space:

"And is there anything else you know…from there?"

"And is there anything else about that [y]?" (when y is a word/phrase your client uses)

"And what kind of [y] is that [y]?"

But do so sparingly! Do not ask these additional CLQs at every space, and do not ask more than one or, at the most, two additional questions. Remember this is meant to be lean; you are not looking to go deeply but to ask just enough to activate the relevant parts of the client's system so that what's neurologically wired to his issue gets included. This helps ensure that any insight or other change that comes about is more likely to be comprehensive and impactful.

Moving the paper or object

The Clean Networks script above directs the client to place the paper or object in a space and then move around it. You can also have the client move the paper or object.

When should you try this? It could be a second round of Clean Networks. If your client struggled to get information or ended his first round confused or with things left unresolved, shifting the goal's position around may help him access some information he could not find from his perspective.

Another clue that a round moving the object could be helpful is if your client personified the goal, that is, attributed personal or humanlike qualities to it. For example, it may have intentions of its own ("It doesn't want this" "It needs that"). Hearing from "it" may prove fruitful.

Of course, you can choose to do this "move the object" version of Clean Networks first or solely as well.

Clean Networks when moving the object script

The questions are essentially the same as what you used above, but this time they are asked about what is written or drawn on the paper or your client's object. Explain to your client before you start that he will be moving the object about and he can stand wherever it seems right for him to be.

Step #1: Establishing the client's want or topic of inquiry

Give *one or both* of these Clean directives:

> **"And draw or write what you would like to have happen...or to know more about."** (gesturing to the paper and markers)

or

> **"And choose an object to represent what would you like to have happen...or to know more about."** (gesturing to your collection of objects or around the space)

Step #2: Setting up

> **"And place that where it seems…right."**

> **"And place yourself where you are in relation to that** (gesturing to the paper or object)**…now."**

Step #3: Gathering Information

When your client is situated, ask:

> **"And what do you know…from there?"**

> **"And what does that** (gesturing to the paper or object) **know…from there?"**

Now repeat this directive and question set about five more times.

> **"And find another space that** (gesturing to the paper or object) **could go to."**

Once your client is satisfied with his new placement of the object, ask:

> **"And what does that** (gesturing to the paper or object) **know…from there?"**

Step #4: Synthesizing

For your final question, direct your client to put the paper or object back in the first space and to stand where he began.

> **"And return that** (gesturing to the paper or object) **to its first space."** (gesturing to its space)

> **"And return to your first space."** (gesturing to the client's first space)

> **"And what do you know from there…now?"**

> **"And what difference…does knowing that…make?"**

FAQs | *Frequently Asked Questions*

How much space will my client need to move about?

There is no set amount of space required. You can work outdoors in a large field or a small garden. You can use an entire room or designate a part of it to use. If space is extremely limited or your client has physical disabilities, he can even define his space as a table top or a piece of paper, using some kind of token to represent himself rather than standing on it. (I usually offer a glass bead with a flat bottom that you get in craft stores. A post-it works too.) As long as your client seems able to "project" himself into or onto the space, any size space will do.

That said, I find most people do best actually moving their whole bodies to different spaces. Being able to look from one area to another seems to help the client embody the sense of different perspectives. If the spaces are very, very close together, some people have difficulty separating their perspectives.

But don't get too hung up on this. Let your client experiment and see what happens. If what he is doing is not working for him and he complains, just nod sagely, look around the space as if considering what else might work, and wait for him to come up with a solution. What you want to avoid is offering your own solution; that wouldn't be Clean!

Do we need anything else besides a space to work in?

You might want to have a pad and pen as well to keep track of a few of the client's key words and to sketch out your client's locations.

Your client may like to have a journal or other paper to write about his experience after the session. Or you could provide some plain paper so he can do a quick "map" of the spaces as a reminder of the session.

How long should a session last?

Times will vary, depending on how much time you have available, your intention, and how you may be incorporating this into other work you are doing with a client. And of course, depending on the experience your client has. You could reasonably conduct a session in as little as 15 minutes with perhaps three or four spaces and for as long as 30 minutes with six spaces.

Is there such a thing as too few or too many spaces?

One determinant as to how many spaces you direct your client to find is how much time you have: the shorter the time, the fewer the spaces you will have. I would suggest a minimum of three, preferably four; fewer than that and your client does not have much of a chance to visit multiple perspectives. If you get more than seven, it may become too much for your client to conceive of as a whole. So as a general rule, try five or six. But be ready to be flexible! Being Clean means being responsive to your client's experience, to what happens in the moment.

What if my client directs me as to where I should stand?

Don't take it personally if your client gestures for or asks you to move during the session. Perhaps you are too close for him to concentrate, too far away for him to feel your attention, or in the way of finding a space. You want to create an atmosphere that empowers your client to self-explore, to determine what he needs in this mysterious, psychoactive space.

How do I know when to go on to the next question?

Pay close attention to your client's nonverbals. If your client is still mentally "working" at a space, do not rush on to the next question. Allow him time to discover what there is to learn. Often clients will look up at you when they are ready.

What if I ask, "And what do you know from there?" and my client repeatedly says, "I don't know" or "I don't know anything?" Maybe this isn't working!

In the FAQ section on Clean Space, I will give you a number of suggestions for how you can handle an "I don't know" response. But for now, let me encourage you to trust your common sense. If over and over your client is not able to access information from spaces, you can switch gears, perhaps changing to another Clean process. No need to make a big announcement that suggests there is a problem or that your client has somehow messed up (yes, some clients will assume this!). Just smoothly segue into an alternative process or mix questions from other processes into your Clean Networks script. For example, Clean Space is similar in many ways to Clean Networks. If your client has gotten some information from some of his Clean Networks spaces, switching to Clean Space may work well because it invites him to revisit those spaces. We are going to be looking at blending different Clean processes' questions further in Section 8.

What if I gesture to a space to return to and my client goes to the wrong spot?

If he does not remember accurately, that's okay. Do not rescue. Do not correct him. If he asks for help, just smile, say nothing, and gesture as if to say, "Wherever seems right." Trust that whatever he comes up with, following his own intuition and knowing will be just right for him.

What if my client says he hasn't found anything of value at the end of a round?

Consider what has emerged for the client. It is possible he may need more than one round of Clean Networks to get to a real breakthrough. Perhaps you will have time to do it in the same session; perhaps it will have to be another time. Just know that because everything is not resolved and wrapped up in a nice bow at the end of this round, it does not mean the Clean process is not working. You will have to assess that with each individual case.

It is not unusual for a breakthrough to be preceded by confusion or a sense of having something "nearly in focus" or "right at your fingertips" but just not having any clarity yet. It can be a good sign, actually. As the mind's container for information on the topic being explored gets fuller and fuller, the mind is pressured to come up with some better, more efficient way of organizing it, of making sense of it all. The act of doing that can lead to new perspectives and new insights. That is the emergent process we have talked about in action.

Ultimately, this is your client's journey. You are not there to *fix* anything or to *change* anything; you are there to facilitate your client's exploration process.

What if my client says he can't remember much of what happened during the session—even right after it ends?

This is not unusual, actually. And it does not seem to bother most clients. Often they will remember only some key piece of information they got that gives them a new perspective or suggests a new direction or action to take, and they are quite satisfied with that. I think what is going on during a session involves an unusually direct connection with the subconscious, and it can be quickly lost to conscious recall, like forgetting a dream shortly after waking up. Forgetting does not mean nothing significant happened.

If your client does seem concerned, you can mention that this is often the case and share the dream comparison. Or rather than "rescue" with an explanation, you could ask a basic Clean Language question:

"And when you can't remember, what would you like to have happen?"

Your client may say, "Oh, it's no big deal," and you will realize nothing more need happen. Or he may say, "I'd like to write it down/do a sketch." Fine. If he asks you to remind him of any of his content, be sure you use only his exact words; add or change nothing!

Whatever he does remember will tell you where his attention is and may help you assess what you will do with the client next.

Finally, if you are only dipping into the chapter here, you may want to check out the FAQs for Clean Space (see pages 67–70), as some are applicable to Clean Networks too.

Example: Vicky

Vicky is very forthcoming. She reports rather matter-of-factly that she was sexually assaulted in a date rape situation about a month ago and that it is her mother's idea that she come to therapy. She slouches in her chair, with arms crossed, looking something between bored and huffy. I start with this CLQ before deciding what process to use.

Facilitator: **And what would you like to have happen…or to know more about?**

Vicky: *Nothing, really. I just need to move on, really. Bad things happen. So it sucks. I can deal with it.*

Now I could start to do all kinds of analyses here and decide what I think Vicky should recognize, what I assume she needs to eventually acknowledge, and so on. Or I can let Vicky do that for herself. I will listen for what she says she wants here and now. I decide to get her moving with a Clean Networks process. She just might be intrigued by working in such an unorthodox manner.

I explain to Vicky how it works and ask whether she is willing to give it a go. She agrees, and I provide several colors of paper and markers.

Facilitator: **And draw or write what you would like to have happen…or to know more about** (gesturing to the paper and markers).

Vicky looks up, a little startled. Perhaps she expected some pushback. She spends a couple of minutes drawing a stick figure of a girl walking, wearing a backpack.

Facilitator: **And place that where it seems…right.**

Vicky puts the paper on the floor in the middle of the room.

Facilitator: **And place yourself where you are in relation to that** (gesturing to the paper) **now.**

Vicky stands about six feet away, facing her drawing.

Facilitator: **And what do you know…from there?**

Vicky: *I know I'm further away from there than I thought. It seems really far away.*

Already, distance from the paper has taken on meaning for Vicky. The space is becoming psycho-activated. I wait while she stares at the picture. I look at the drawing too, content with having no idea what she is thinking right now. She appears inner focused, not paying attention to me at all. Finally, I go on.

Facilitator: **And is there anything else you know…from there?**

Vicky: *I notice I have a backpack.*

She focuses on a metaphor: the backpack. Vicky didn't give much information. But it seemed significant enough to her to mention it, so I hold her attention there a bit longer with another CLQ.

Facilitator: **And is there anything else about** that backpack?

Vicky: *Yes. I sense it's important, but I don't know why or what's in it.*

I do not let myself get pulled into trying to fix this, to see what I can do to solve the mystery. Especially if she has experienced a trauma, a client may not know something she is not ready to know, and I do not want to rush her or even suggest that she has to know. This is where the panning for gold processes can be so helpful; you strive to move at the client's rate of readiness and keep her moving so she is less likely to get stuck in an emotionally wrenching place. I stick to the process and keep Vicky moving.

Facilitator: **And find another space.**

Vicky moves back two steps.

Facilitator: **And what do you know…from there?**

Vicky: *From here, I can see the backpack is holding me back. It's a* back *pack; a pack that's holding me back.*

Again, I wait quietly, giving Vicky all the time she seems to want to spend there. When she seems satisfied, I ask:

Facilitator: **And find another space.**

This time Vicky moves to the other side of the room and faces away from her first two spaces.

Facilitator: **And what do you know…from there?**

Vicky: *I feel older in this space, like older and wiser, somehow. From here, I know that backpack is holding me back, but it also has stuff in it that I need to take with me, things that will help me when I move on.*

Because Vicky had started the session sounding rather angry and dismissive, I do not want to take the chance of triggering defensiveness by digging too deeply. I let her system come to its own realizations.

Facilitator: **And find another space.**

Vicky moves to a chair and sits on the floor beside it, leaning her head up against it. Suddenly, she doesn't look like a defiant teenager, but a little girl.

Facilitator: **And what do you know…from there?**

Vicky: *I can't put it into words, really. I feel sort of protected, with this chair to lean on. I could hide behind it if I wanted to.*

Vicky closes her eyes, and I do not rush her. Perhaps she wants to go behind the chair, but I do not suggest it. I stick to the script.

Facilitator: **And find another space.**

Vicky gets up and starts walking around, stopping, starting again, seeming to search for a place that holds some information. Eventually she settles in a space in a part of the room she has not been in yet, again about six feet from her drawing. And then, before I can speak, Vicky does.

Vicky: *I'm uncomfortable here. Do I have to stay here?*

I make another judgment call. I do not want Vicky to get overwhelmed, but then managing to hang in there when feeling uncomfortable long enough to deal with what presents itself can be part of any healing process. She does not look panicky or convey a sense of not feeling safe. So I ask just one question, keeping my voice calm and neutral.

Facilitator: **And what do you know…from there?**

Vicky: *I know I don't like this feeling and I want to move. And I'm going to.*

She spoke with conviction. I merely nod and direct:

Facilitator: **And find another space.**

Vicky goes back to the chair, this time standing on the other side.

Facilitator: **And what do you know…from there?**

Vicky: *I know that just knowing this chair is here to lean on or sit in or hide behind is enough* (as she nods repeatedly).

Facilitator: **And return to your first space** (gesturing to the space). **And what do you know from there…now?**

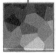

She points to her drawing.

Vicky: *Can I move closer?*

I nod and gesture toward the drawing, with a slight shrug as if to say, "It's up to you. Sure."

Vicky halves her distance from the drawing. I repeat:

Facilitator: **And what do you know from there...now?**

Vicky: *From here, now, I know my mother is just trying to help me. Bringing me here is one of her ways of doing that. Before, I sort of thought she was punishing me. But I guess I'm okay with it now...I get it...I get it. Okay.*

And she looks up and moves back to her original chair, sits, and fools with something in her purse, clearly signaling she is done.

Here she is at the end of her session, and it is the first time Vicky has mentioned her mother. Was she thinking about her all along? Was it a connection that emerged at the end? What does a backpack and a chair and spaces offering different perspectives have to do with the insight Vicky came to? What exactly is it she "gets"? What's "okay" now? I could ask more questions, but would that be the most helpful thing for Vicky right now?

Vicky did not appear to need to go through a lot of cognitive processing to get to her insight, and I do not need to get her to analyze it for it to be meaningful for her. She came in sounding guarded, and I do not want to suggest she has to share what she doesn't want to. I go no further.

How will I know if the session helped? She may tell me outright. I might also be able to tell by what her identified want is in her next session. Her attitude then may tell me as well, for it sounds like what happened may open her to accepting my help...and her mother's...in a way she evidently wasn't before.

That is the wisdom of the client's system: to know this was the first thing she needed to deal with, for without a willingness to accept help, how much were the sessions likely to accomplish? But then, that is my take on what might have happened for Vicky. I can make all the educated guesses I like about what Vicky's spaces and descriptions meant, but ultimately they will be assumptions. I have to settle for not knowing for sure.

Remember, Clean questions are about helping your client discover more about herself, for empowering *self-exploration*, not asking for *self-explanation*. Metaphors and spatial experiences work in mysterious ways. Embrace the mystery.

PROCESS #6: CLEAN SPACE

Designed to:

    Clarify any issue or topic

    Open a client to new perspectives and possibilities regarding his issue

Useful for:

    Considering one thing from multiple perspectives

    Comparing options

    Establishing priorities

    Making decisions

    Loosening up old patterns

    Revealing hidden issues and connections between issues

Time to allot: about 45 minutes

Materials needed:

    Post-its and a pen or markers, preferably in a choice of colors

    Optional: masking tape, a collection of objects to choose from or an object your client brings to represent his topic of inquiry

Clean Space is the first of Grove's spatial processes and the one from which his Emergent Knowledge techniques evolved (Harland, 2009). The more Grove experimented, the more he simplified his spatial techniques. So this first one is a bit more involved than Clean Networks. But I think there are times and situations when Clean Space is very useful. You will be glad to have it in your toolbox, and it is not difficult to master.

The Clean Space process

With a Clean Space process, the client and the space are really doing the work. You, the facilitator, use a fairly simple script consisting of a limited number of questions and directing statements. They guide the client to map out a landscape of spaces, as with Clean Networks. This time, the client marks each space with a post-it so he can return to it. As he revisits his spaces, your CLQs ask him to consider what he knows from there about his *other* spaces. His very movements help create new connections between these various ideas and feelings, weaving a web of interrelationships. With new connections come new perspectives; greater clarity; new concepts; and perhaps, new feelings, thoughts, and goals.

Frankly, the Clean Space process seems more about creating a network than Clean Networks does, which makes the names somewhat mystifying to me. But I appreciate that the processes developed over time. Had they been created and titled simultaneously, the names given them might have better suited their distinguishing characteristics. We have inherited David Grove's nomenclature, and it is well established in the Clean community now. I do not foresee it changing, whatever its shortcomings.

Clean Space script[6]

Step #1: Establishing the client's want or topic of inquiry [x]

"And draw or write what you would like to have happen…or know more about" (gesturing to the paper and markers).

or

"And choose an object to represent what would you like to have happen…or to know more about" (gesturing to your collection of objects or around the space).

Step #2: Setting up

"And place that where it seems…right."

"And place yourself where you are in relation to that (gesturing to the paper/ object)**…now."**

Step #3: Gathering information

"And what do you know…from there?"

"And what do you know from there…about that?" (gesturing to the paper/object)

After your client has collected information from the space—not before!—invite him to name the space and label it. Why wait until he is finished in that space? Why not start with the naming? Because it takes answering your questions for your client to learn what there is to learn from a space. He does not know that when he first arrives. Help him discover and experience that new information before putting a label on it.

"And what could that space be called?"

"And put that down." (gesturing to the post-its and marker)

"And mark that space." (gesturing to the space)

Even though you now have a name to call that space by, be sure you also gesture toward it when you refer to it, as the space itself and not just the name holds information.

From here, you will have the client identify about five more spaces, as you did in Clean Networks, with the directive:

"And find another space."

"And what do you know…from there?"

"And what do you know from there…about [x]**?"** (gesturing to the paper/object)

Then you repeat this pattern of one directive and two questions until your client has identified six spaces in all.

Step #4: Revisiting spaces

This next step is where Clean Space diverges most significantly from Clean Networks. You are going to be weaving a web of interconnections between the spaces by revisiting each one and asking what is known from there about some of the other spaces.

"And return to [name of the space]**."** (gesturing to the space)

Once the client is settled, ask:

"And what do you know from there…now?"

"And what do you know from there… about [name of space]**?"** (gesture toward another space)

Not clear on how this would work? The goal here is to revisit all the spaces at least once and to try to connect each space with several other spaces, time permitting.

Example:

Client stands on   Facilitator asks about

#1...........................#3, #5, #2
#6...........................#4, #1, topic of inquiry
#2...........................#4, #3, #5
#5...........................#2, #3, #1
#4...........................#1, #5, topic of inquiry
#3...........................#2, #4, #6

Notice that asking what a client knows *from* Space #2 *about* Space #5 is not the same thing as asking what he knows *from* Space #5 *about* Space #2.

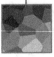

Pairing spaces

With five or six spaces, the possible pairings of spaces grow so much that you cannot reasonably get to them all in the time constraints of a typical session. Be sure your client visits each space at least once. From there, you will have to choose which other spaces to ask about, being sure to include them all at some time. Careful attention to the logic of your client's exploration will suggest which pairings are likely to prove fruitful for the client. But sometimes pairings that simply come up as you check off the list will yield surprising results, so watch out for your assumptions.

Grove referred to spaces that hold more new or helpful information as "sweet spots." Return your client to them or ask about them from other spaces often. I have noticed clients frequently have a place that offers a "higher perspective" (and, not surprisingly, the client often wants to get *up* on something or place the post-it higher than the others); this is often a place of great wisdom.

The fundamental idea here is that it is in the connections between the spaces that significant new information can likely be uncovered. That is why you do not develop extensive information from any one space but rather to keep the client moving and experiencing the *relationships between* the pieces of information/spaces. Often the client comes away with detailed information that the individual spaces hold *and* a new vision of the whole.

Step #5: Synthesizing

Once you have finished having your client revisit spaces, direct:

> **"And return to** [name of Space #1]**"** (gesturing to space).

> **"And when all that** (gesturing around the entire psychoactive space), **what do you know from there…now?"**

> **"And what do you know from there now…about** [x]**?"** (gesturing to goal/topic)

Finally, invite him to take this knowing out into his world by asking:

> **"And what difference…does knowing that…make?"** (all-inclusive gesture)

When the session is done, invite your client to pick up his post-its himself. They will hold emotional meaning for him, so it is better that he picks them up rather than you. Some clients want to keep the notes; others do not care. Some will dramatically choose to throw one particular post-it away or rip it to pieces! Who is to say what meaning these pieces of paper now hold for your client? Be respectful of them by not touching them.

Post-session options

Invite the client to make a sketch/map of the locations of his post-its before picking them up. You can suggest he may want to lay them out at a later time and work with them more on his own.

Your client may wish to spend some time writing down some of the information he developed during the session or responding to the experience in some other way. Or you may want to segue into facilitating with another technique or activity here. We will get to some possibilities in a later section.

Often, after a client has finished, he may be talking in a typical conversational manner, but some inner integration of this experience is still going on. Remember: stay Clean! Don't interpret, analyze, or give advice.

Clean Space option

Choosing a word for the client

Sometimes you may want to ask your client to find a space that holds more information about a particular word. Perhaps it is a word that your client suggests has a space, one that he has either pointed to, looked at, or mentions.

Example:

Client: *I've got a lot of family support backing me up* (looking behind himself).

Facilitator: **And find a space that knows about** family support backing you up.

In all likelihood, the client will find a space behind his back.

Or you could choose a particular word your client mentions that stands out and seems worth exploring, given what your client has been talking about. I do not encourage you to do this with every space because generally you are better off trusting your client to decide what to explore next. But once in a while, you may feel the logic of your client's experience calls for more information about a particular word. Experiment…and be ready to abandon the practice if what you choose does not appear to be helpful to your client. Remember: the session is not about satisfying your curiosity. Nor is it about you as an experienced professional deciding what a client with this type of issue should be concerned about. Think Clean, which means keeping a watchful eye out for your assumptions and leaving your client in charge of the content of his session.

FAQs | *Frequently Asked Questions*

Do I need to do any prepping of my client if he's done Clean Networks before?

If your client has done Clean Networks, you may want to explain before you start that Clean Space is similar but has some differences, namely that he will be naming each space and marking it with a post-it because he is going to be coming back to it. You can just say something like "You will be doing another go-round of the spaces." You don't have to get into what you will be asking that is different at this point.

Why name the spaces? Isn't it easier to just refer to spaces as "there"?

There is less for you to track if the client does not name spaces, and you can choose to work that way. But this is one instance where I have opted not to stay as lean as possible.

I am convinced that the invitation to name the space invites emergence. It does not always happen as you would expect because emergence is unpredictable by nature. Sometimes the client selects a word or short phrase that has come up in his description of what he knows from the space to be the name; it does not suggest a new level or order of meaning. Sometimes, however, the name the client settles on transcends the content of what he has described so far, or it seems to. I have often heard clients make an unexpected leap. For example, a client may have talked about this place being "uncomfortable" and of "not knowing a lot about [the topic] from here," and when asked to name it, he will say "Home" or "Familiar," names that seem to imply new and often broader associations. Perhaps he was aware of them all along, and it is only now that I am hearing about them. Or perhaps, as he searched for a word that encompassed all he knew about that space, a new way of organizing the information emerged. He is categorizing it differently.

When a higher order name emerges, the same thing has happened on a micro-scale that the Clean Space process is looking to have happen on a larger scale. In the example above, it is with the bits of information collected in *one* space that a new organizing pattern emerged. The same could happen in other spaces. And it could happen with the information collected from all the spaces—reintegrating into one grand, new whole.

What if my client wants to place a post-it somewhere that can't be reached or is dangerous?

After very briefly explaining the problem, invite your client to find a space that "can stand in for that [inaccessible space]." Basically, you are having him locate a surrogate space. Personally, I have never had a client baulk at this.

What if my client wants to move a label?

As your client's understanding of the way he organizes his perception of his world expands, changes may well happen. Allow your client to move the label and explore what happens when it is in its new location with a round of questions. One such shift in the system may result in major changes elsewhere.

What if my client wants to change the name of a space?

Follow his lead. If he wants to change the name of the space, it is because he has some new understanding to explore. Once he has written down the name, ask "And what do you know from there *now*?" It has a new characteristic and will likely have new information to convey.

What if my client starts directing himself?

If your client is familiar with the Clean Space process, he may well take over and suggest his own next space or begin moving himself between spaces. Good! He is not challenging your authority; he is *self-modeling*, creating a model of his own inner landscape.

Honor that knowing, while also assuring the client does not leave out potentially important information by returning him periodically to any neglected (unvisited) spaces when you get to the revisiting phase. Your client may most need you to keep in mind the very things he habitually overlooks, avoids, or rushes through!

And if you have an experienced client who is doing a fine job facilitating himself? Feel like you are not being useful? Wonder how you can justify charging such a client? Don't underestimate the power of your holding that space for your client, of keeping the focus, of offering acceptance and empathy. You *are* serving your client.

What if my client starts to get highly emotional or upset at a space? Should I move him on quickly or avoid returning him there?

Not necessarily. Just because we began by focusing on wants rather than problems does not mean problems or negative thoughts or feelings will not come up; they may well have the potential to yield meaningful information or experiences. You need not be thrown by a few tears or expressions of discomfort.

That said, use your own good judgment. Naturally, if a client is on the verge of a panic attack, you do not have to be rigid about insisting he visit or stay in a space! If he flat out says he doesn't want to go to a space, do not push him to do so. You could suggest he find another space that "knows something about [name of the space he does not want to visit]." Getting some distance from the space can help the client learn from it without being overwhelmed by it.

What if I ask "And what do you know from there?" and my client says "I don't know" or "I don't know anything"?

I know I said I was going to keep this book simple, but this issue invites lots of interesting potential responses I just can't resist sharing with you. If it is too much for you at this point when you have so much to absorb, just pick one or two responses to have ready and leave it at that. Come back at a later time when you are more experienced and add some of these other Clean questions and phrases taken from other processes to your repertoire.

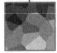

First of all, do not abandon the process at the first "I don't know." Often it simply means "I don't know yet." Wait quietly and patiently; just nod and direct your gaze and energy to the space where he is standing. Do not engage your client's eyes; you do not want to encourage him to look to you for the answer. You could say,

> **"Take all the time you need."**

A client who is new to Clean Space or to working with you may need reassurance that his session is perfectly normal. This simple directive gives him permission to slow down and just let the answer come. He may be feeling he should have an answer immediately and rush himself. Express no impatience or concern. Even if your client is not finding the answer to the question you asked, you can be sure plenty is still going on for him as long as he is focused on himself and not on how you are responding.

Notice his body language; you will likely be able tell if he is puzzling out an answer or has abandoned hope of doing so. If you have waited and your client is looking at you expectantly with a look in his eye that suggests he is not exploring his inner experience anymore, you can speak again.

Nod knowingly, suggesting this is perfectly normal, and simply ask **"And what could that space be called?"** The client may name it "I don't know" or something else entirely. Treat it just as you would any other space; perhaps when he returns to it later, he will discover something else.

If I facilitate another session with this client on the same topic of inquiry, should I direct him to reuse the same post-its in the same locations?

The ending of any session is somewhat arbitrary, as the entire system of spaces and the information they hold is dynamic and constantly in motion. For this reason, I recommend you start over. While your client may elect to use the same post-it or object to describe or represent his want or topic of inquiry, the rest of his system will likely have changed in response to his first session, so start fresh and see what emerges.

On the other hand, if your client puts his post-its back where they were, do not stop or correct him; honor his knowing. So where would you begin? Once his post-its are back in place, start with the second directive in Step #2, **"And place yourself where you are in relation that…now"** (gesturing to the paper/object), followed by **"And what do you know from there?"**

Then be ready to respond creatively to how your client wants to work with his spaces. It may not go exactly as scripted, and it is your job to adjust, not your client's. You could have your client start revisiting his spaces, finding out what he knows now. He may want to move his spaces or change their names. He may realize he wants to consider a new want or topic from the same spaces. He may find his insight or conclusions have evolved. He will adjust to the changes in his internal system and knowing, and your role is to facilitate a session that allows him to do that.

How can I tell whether anything helpful is happening for my client?

Sometimes it is obvious: your client will excitedly tell you a positive shift has occurred. Or the information he discovers is clearly relevant or beneficial and/or offers new insights. Other times, the session starts some change in motion that will become clear only after—possibly long after—the session is over.

If your client is readily finding spaces, getting information from them, and engrossed with the process, then rest easy he is getting something out of the experience. Trust the process and trust your client.

Finally, you may want to review the FAQs from Clean Networks (see pages 55–57), as many are applicable to Clean Space too.

Example: Jaime (continued)

We continue here with Jaime's session, which we began with a Clean Start (see page 32). You will notice that a couple of the questions or directives I give are variations or options. They demonstrate how I adjust the process to what my client says and does. Yes, there is a script, but you need to stay on your toes, responding to what comes up.

We left off with:

Facilitator: **And what do you know…from there?**

Jaime: *I don't know that I know anything. I'm sort of at a loss.*

Directing my gaze to the post-it with *career* on it and gesturing toward it…

Facilitator: **And what do you know from there…about** career?

Jaime: *This is where I am now, facing "career." It just seems like one big, humongous question looming at me. My mind's a blank!*

If you are new to Clean Space, you might be panicking about now. You might wonder whether Clean Space is "working." But getting a "blank mind" or an "I don't know" *is* an answer. Just stick with the process. Something more always happens!

I wait until Jaime looks back at me, signaling she has finished considering the space for now.

Facilitator: **And what could this space be called?**

Jaime: *This space is called "Question" (Space #1).*

Facilitator: **And put that down.** (gesturing to the pad of post-its) **And mark that space** (gesturing to the space on which she is standing). **And find another space.**

After wandering around the room a bit, Jaime selects another space and looks up.

Facilitator: **And what do you know…from there?**

Jaime: *This space feels sort of scary. The unknown feels like this enormous space.*

Facilitator: **And what do you know from there…about career?**

Jaime: *I feel like I'm standing still, confused. All my friends are apparently seeing roads when all I see is a big, open, unmarked space. I like my safe little walls, thank you very much!*

Facilitator: **And is there anything else you know…from there?**

Jaime: *It's oppressive. I feel so weighted down by the unknowns.*

Facilitator: **And what could this space be called?**

Jaime: *This space is called "Unknown" (Space #2).*

I nod toward the post-it note pad, inviting Jaime to write that down. Once she's done, I add,

Facilitator: **And mark that space. And find another space.**

Jaime wanders around until she selects a space. Once she settles in, I ask:

Facilitator: **And what do you know…from there?**

Jaime: *From here I know I can continue to work for a year after graduating at the college's theater. It's run by professionals, and I can continue to be a set-design grunt.*

Facilitator: **And is there anything else you know…from there?**

Jaime: *It'll be good! I'll keep learning, maybe make some connections. Dilemma solved!*

Facilitator: **And what could this space be called?**

Jaime: *This space is called "More of the Same" (Space #3).*

Jaime doesn't wait for my prompt to write the word down and place the post-it on the spot where she is standing. But I notice as she writes, her expression changes; she doesn't seem as pleased as she was just seconds ago.

I could continue to give an open-ended invitation to find more spaces, or I could be more directive. In the moment, her change of expression nudges me to guide Jaime to explore something she just said.

Facilitator: **And find a space that knows something about** keep learning.

Jaime climbs on top of a coffee table.

Facilitator: **And what do you know…from there?**

Jaime: *This space feels really open and spacious!* (Jaime spreads her arms out and rotates side to side, smiling.) *I'm not really getting any information or suggestions here, like set design or something; mostly it's just a feeling!*

I find it is not unusual for clients to find a space that is higher than the others; they climb on chairs, tables, stone walls, etc. My sense from what clients find there is that these are spaces offering a higher or broader perspective and often seem to hold information that clients find particularly helpful. In this case, I ask a Clean Language question to help Jaime develop a more specific description, since it sounds like this feeling of hers could be a resource.

Facilitator: **And what kind of** feeling **is that** feeling?

Jaime: *Like I'm filled with energy! Sort of free and open and alive!*

Facilitator: **And what could this space be called?**

Jaime: *This is "Possibilities"* (Space #4).

Facilitator: **And put that down. And mark that space. And find another space.**

Jaime moves about until she is near the bookcase.

Facilitator: **And what do you know…from there?**

Jaime: *This space is full of supposed to's. Like I should know what I want to do. And I should know where I want to live. My parents would never say it, but I know they would really like me to move back to my hometown. It would really disappoint them if I left. But maybe I should set sail, you know, move to New York or somewhere. Ooh…that feels scary to say out loud.*

Facilitator: **And what could this space be called?**

Jaime: *"Expectations"* (Space #5).

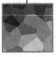

Jaime writes it down and marks her spot. She has now established five spaces. With my eye on the clock, I will stop having Jaime add more spaces and move to Step #3: reconsidering spaces from the perspective of another space. For no particular reason, as she will revisit them all, I start with Space #4, from where I ask about Space #3.

Facilitator:	**And return to** Possibilities. **And what do you know from there…now?**

Jaime:	*It feels more open now.*

Facilitator:	**And what do you know from there…about** More of the Same? (gesturing to Space #3)

Jaime:	*Oh! From up here* (on the coffee table), *I realize I can't stay at the college theater, not really. It's* (laughs, as if at herself)…*more of the same. It's safe and comfortable, but I have to spread my wings. Time to move on.*

This seems like an aha! moment, and you might think it is a natural place to end the session. But I stick to the Clean Space structure and continue directing Jaime's attention to other spaces. Keeping her at Space #4, I ask about Space #1 now.

Facilitator:	**And what do you know from there…about** Question? (gesturing to Space #1)

Jaime:	*I realize there are infinite possibilities I could apply my art and creativity to! I can be like an explorer. Explorers don't know what they're going to find…they go into uncharted territory to see what they discover.*

Facilitator:	**And what do you know from there about** Expectations? (gesturing to Space #5)

Jaime:	*It's like I'm in a crow's nest of a ship. I can see over those expectations. They seemed so big when I was there, but from here, they seem…not just little, but not even real.*

I do not rush Jaime. I wait while she mulls this insight over until she looks back at me, ready to go on.

Facilitator:	**And return to** More of the Same (gesturing to Space #3). **And what do you know from there…now?**

Jaime:	*When I was here before, it felt good, but now it feels sort of lifeless, like the wind is out of the sails.*

Facilitator:	**And is there anything else about that** wind?

Jaime:	*Yes, it is blowing in another direction now…toward Possibilities, actually.*

As Jaime's attention has moved to Possibilities, I ask about that next.

Facilitator: **And what do you know from there…about** Possibilities? (gesturing to Space #4)

Jaime: *The wind is what energizes possibilities into reality. I have to pay attention to which way the wind is blowing.*

Facilitator: **And what do you know from there…about career?** (gesturing to topic of inquiry space)

Jaime: *That I don't have to find a permanent answer to my question; I can be open to possibilities! I can keep readjusting my sails.*

Facilitator: **And what do you know from there…about** Unknown? (gesturing to Space #2)

Jaime: *Nothing more, really.*

By now, you can see why you will probably want to keep a list of the numbers of spaces, checking them off to make sure you get to each one at least once.

Facilitator: **And return to Unknown** (gesturing to Space #2). **And what do you know from there…now?**

Jaime: *Huh! It doesn't feel so scary now.*

Facilitator: **And what do you know from there…about** Question? (gesturing to Space #1)

Jaime: *It's okay that I don't know what career to embark on or even what questions to ask.*

Facilitator: **And what do you know from there…about** Possibilities? (gesturing to Space #4)

Jaime: *That it's about getting out there and trying new things, talking to people, getting ideas. It's about an attitude of being excited to embrace the unknown.*

Facilitator: **And what do you know from there…about** More of the Same? (gesturing to Space #3)

Jaime: *I know I have a way sometimes of falling back into helplessness, where I feel like a kid. And I know from here that I don't have to let that happen. I can connect with Possibilities (and she turns to face Space #4).*

Jaime had just considered Possibilities from this space with the question before this one, but as she has turned back to face it again, I check to see whether there is something more for her there. Or perhaps she simply wants to sense its energy again.

Facilitator: **And is there anything else you know from there…about** Possibilities? (gesturing to Space #4)

Jaime: *Not really. It just feels good to face it! Like I can drink in the feeling if I face it.*

I pause, giving Jaime time to drink it in.

Facilitator: **And what do you know from there…about** Expectations? (gesturing to Space #5)

Jaime: *It's like I arbitrarily decided these things are expected of me. Where did I come up with them?*

Facilitator: **And return to** Expectations (gesturing to Space #5). **And what do you know from there…now?**

Jaime: *I was putting up false walls.*

Facilitator: **And what do you know from there…about Question** (gesturing to Space #1)?

Jaime: *I know that the information in this space is not what's going to help me answer my question. Staying here is not going to help me now.*

Facilitator: **And what do you know from there…about** Unknown (gesturing to Space #2)**?**

Jaime: *That I don't need to compare myself to what my friends are doing. It's okay that I don't know where I'm headed right now.*

Jaime has now revisited Spaces 2–5, and it is time to send her back to her original starting place. It held the perspective she came into our session with today, and returning there will give her a chance to experience how her thinking and/or feelings have changed.

Facilitator: **And return to** Question (gesturing to Space #1).
And when all that (gesturing to all the spaces), **what do you know from there…now?**

Jaime: *I feel much better than when I started!*

Facilitator: **And what do you know from there about** career? (gesturing to the paper)

Jaime: *I know I don't have to find the career I'll do for the rest of my life. I don't have to know the whole path.*

Facilitator: **And what difference...does knowing that...make?**

Jaime: *I feel a huge sense of relief, like it's going to be okay. Phew! All I need to know is the next step. Like any explorer worthy of the name! It's like I'm remembering that...not discovering it. Like I'd forgotten...I feel sort of silly that I got myself so worked up.*

I expect that to many observers, it would seem as if Jaime is getting messages from several spaces that are essentially the same, particularly as she reconsiders spaces for the second and third time. It is as if the information from different perspectives is converging into one coherent whole. This often (but not always) happens; one dominant message begins to be reinforced from multiple points of view.

One of the things I like about Clean Space is how readily it reminds both client and facilitator to hold our assumptions for the session lightly, for what message ends up shining through loud and clear may not be at all what either of us expected. We might, for example, have thought Jaime's message would have been about a specific career choice for her. How wrong we would have been! Using this Clean process circumvented our expectations and opened the door to Jaime's productive exploration.

As it turned out, Jaime didn't take the safe, familiar job at her college. She moved to New York with friends without a job waiting, scrambled for a while, tried different things, and a year later, went back to school for a degree in interior design. She is happily employed in that field today. She found her calling not by taking a personality or career inventory test but by deciding to become an explorer.

I connected with Jaime again just recently and asked her what she recalled about her Clean Space experience 10 years ago. She wrote me back in detail. I think her (abbreviated) answer is worth sharing so you can get a sense of what a Clean experience can be like for a client, how significant shifts can just happen, and what a difference they can make.

Jaime: *I don't remember a lot of the specifics of the session. I remember the physicality of the session—moving around a lot, climbing on things...I see now what a big difference there was between my two perceptions of the big open space, scary when I thought I had to be able to navigate the whole thing, but then invigorating and liberating when I realized I didn't. Just a perception shift. I gave myself permission to keep believing what I always had before: that life is long, and each thing you do is a success as long as you learn something new that you can apply to the next step. Up on the coffee table, I realized I had lost sight of it with all the graduation hubbub. I had constructed these parameters for myself that had no relation to my usual M.O.. It did feel like those parameters had been very flimsy, once I let them go. Once they were down...it really did just feel kind of silly that I had ever thought they were real.*

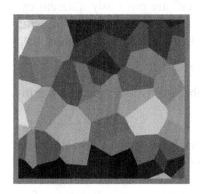

Section Four

When the Page Becomes Psychoactive

WORKING WITH METAPHORS

I have discussed metaphors and Grove's reasoning for working with them in Section 1. We are going to revisit them now and consider more Grovian methods for exploring them. But first, to review…

> A metaphor: one thing is equated to a decidedly different thing to clarify the nature of the first thing's traits or qualities. Often metaphors compare an abstract concept or feeling with a tangible object.

To explain to someone else what it feels like to be depressed, an individual may call upon a more concrete experience the listener can more likely imagine or identify with. For example, while suffering from depression and "being in a well" are obviously different experiences in many ways, for some individuals, they share feelings characteristic of being trapped in some deep, dark place that is hopelessly difficult to get out of. So metaphors help us communicate with one another.

What Grove's work with clients demonstrates is that metaphors serve an even more significant purpose in a person's inner world.

As a client accesses and describes his internalized metaphors, he reveals his subconscious's encoded representation of his experiences, beliefs, and theories about how to survive and manage in his world as he conceives it. His mind/body system, with all its strengths and weaknesses, insights and confusions, wisdom and maladaptations, approaches the surface of conscious awareness where it can learn from itself, heal, and grow.

To put it another way using another metaphor, you help your client pull up some of his subconscious metaphor files and sort through, rearrange, delete, merge, add to, and otherwise improve them. He then tucks his metaphor files back into his subconscious. His mind/body system opens the appropriate file again when he needs help making sense of his world, determining how to respond to events, feelings, and making daily decisions.

When his inner experience is expressed in a tangible form, the client is given something to engage with, something that has characteristics of objects that obey the laws of his system's logic. A metaphor may move, grow, or melt. Perhaps it wants or needs protection or freeing. Whatever its qualities and its story, it is now accessible to be known and, possibly, changed when before it was not.

David Grove developed the first of his Clean methodologies, Clean Language, to work with such client-generated metaphors, magnifying the power of metaphor therapy with his Clean concept.

Change the metaphor, change the self

It gives your client a surprising sense of connecting with his innermost self when he finds these internalized metaphors. Often, it is just what he needs to resolve the dilemmas that bring him to you as his old strategies and patterns come to light. He discovers new possibilities and makes different choices. Sometimes such choices and changes happen subconsciously; the client simply reports that "something" has shifted and what was a problem now seems manageable. There is no need for interpretation of the metaphors—not by you nor by the client. The new perspective or solution *emerges* on its own.

But clarity about one's metaphors doesn't always resolve problems. For example, a metaphor that once served a useful purpose may have outlived its usefulness, and yet the client's system is still guided by it. Discovering it doesn't always make it go away or restructure itself. There is more you can do with Clean Language and metaphors that we will not be covering with these 12 lean Clean processes (see Campbell, 2012, 2013). For now, should such a problematic metaphor reveal itself, remember: you are *panning for gold*, collecting information and then letting the client's subconscious system work with it. Just allow the problem to be acknowledged and keep on. You may choose to address it with another methodology or technique *after the Clean session is completed*. Just be sure you remain Clean with regard to the information that came out during the Clean session; because it comes from such an open, vulnerable place, it should command an almost sacred respect.

Metaphor landscapes and metaphor maps

In Clean lingo, as a number of metaphors with relationships to one another amass, we refer to them as a client's *metaphor landscape*. A physical representation of the metaphor landscape is called a *metaphor map*. If you have had an opportunity to be a Clean facilitator or client with one of the spatial processes we have covered so far, you have experienced how significant the location of an object or of oneself can be. You can see why the use of the term *map* for a physicalization of the metaphors is so appropriate.

Drawings elicit metaphors

One of the ways Grove had a client physicalize and explore his metaphors was to have him draw. When a client depicts what something "is like" for him or what he would like it to be like, he has no option but to use metaphors. Having to select a few lines, colors, and/or images, he has to be giving only an impression of what it (whatever *it* is) is similar to. In making the picture, he creates symbols or images that put what may be intangible or has been in a nonverbal state into concrete form.

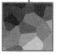

Advantages of drawings

1. Where things are located in space in relation to one another can hold and communicate massive amounts of information. A drawing automatically reveals it.

2. A drawing keeps the whole of the client's landscape in front of him. When things are simply spoken, what was said a few minutes ago can easily drift out of the client's awareness. But when he has drawn at least some elements on the page, they serve as reminders. This is true for the facilitator as well: your client's drawing makes it easier for you to remember your client's metaphor landscape. If you are new to Clean Language, this can be a big help!

3. There are times when a client's feelings threaten to overwhelm him or confuse him because they are conflicted. He may struggle with such feelings and accompanying thoughts as they come to conscious awareness; he may not be ready to verbalize them aloud. By drawing what he knows, the client is able to step away from what emerges: it "lives on the page" for a time where he can see it without having to quite "be in it." Just as moving about in space can help your client consider his inner world from different perspectives, so too looking at a drawing of symbols of that inner world can provide distance and perspective.

Drawings can trigger "art anxiety"

Be prepared for clients who worry that their pictures will be judged "not good enough." I make a point of letting my clients know that stick figures are fine, that abstract pictures of just colors or circles or whatever are fine. I assure them that they will get to keep their own metaphor maps and that they don't have to show them to anyone unless they want to!

I find a little gentle humor helps. Letting reluctant clients know that my metaphor map drawings are laughable seems to have relieved many. My intent in telling them this is to let them know (1) I make these drawings too and that (2) I am not one to be judging the maps for artistic merit.

Also the words you choose to invite your client to draw will depend on your individual client and your context. An art therapist may have no qualms calling the picture a drawing, for example. If art therapy is not your field, you may want to refer to it as a *sketch* or even a *metaphor map*. By avoiding the words "drawing" or "picture," the art phobia many clients have may be sidestepped.

And if your client still resists drawing? I suggest using another Clean process. Your client is telling you that for whatever reason, he does not feel right about drawing. Trust his knowing. He may change his mind later. And with more experience with Clean processes, he just might get curious.

FACILITATING TIPS

Preparing your client

How you set up your contract with your client as to what he wants and can expect from the session and from you will vary depending on your profession. You probably already have a system worked out to determine and explain all this.

In terms of Clean drawing processes, you will direct your client's attention to explore his drawing, looking at both details and the whole. (Envision working a video camera that shows where your client's attention goes. You would be *zooming in* for close-ups and *zooming out* for panoramic views.) You will do this by giving short directives and asking simple questions, in some cases sticking pretty closely to a script that varies little regardless of what your client says. Your client may add to or change his drawing as he discovers more information.

So what should you say to your client? Of course, you should put this in your own words, but perhaps I can help. In addition to the suggestions on page 20, here is an idea of the sort of things you might want to say to your client to prepare him for the drawing processes in this section.

> "What we're going to do is probably a different way of exploring a goal or topic you want to know more about than you may have tried before. It's quite simple, really. I'm going to ask you to do a sketch of your topic. Stick figures are fine! Doodles are fine. This doesn't have to be about making a beautiful work of art.

> "Then, I'll ask some simple questions. There are no right or wrong answers; this is about your noticing more about your topic. I may repeat some of your words back to you to give you a chance to explore them further. You'll very likely discover you know more about your topic than you realized. You can add to or change your drawing as you go. At the end of the session, the sketch is yours to keep.

> "The session will probably take about ____ minutes, and then we'll have some time to talk about what you discovered and what you would like to have happen, if you're open to that. Any questions before we begin?"

Whatever it is you decide to say, prepare your explanation ahead of time. Without one, you may find your client baulks at what seem like odd or unusual questions or repeatedly interrupts his process to clarify what is expected. And there is the chance that you will find yourself blithering away trying to explain it all, which will surely detract from creating a calm, focused environment where your client's metaphor map is the center of his attention.

Hands off the drawing

Just as the space a client wanders in becomes psychoactive, so does the paper on which he draws. As metaphors begin to populate the page and the metaphor landscape reveals itself, they take on emotional significance. Just as you should not walk across the psychoactive space a client is actively engaged with, so you should not touch his drawing. *Gesture toward it*; pointing and touching can feel intrusive.

Pacing

Notice the pauses (…marked with dots…) between the words of some of these questions. They are very important. You want your client to search for his answers from an intuitive place of knowing, not a cognitive, assessing sort of place. To help this process, Grove's trance-inducing wording and pacing is very helpful. The best way to get a feel for how slowly to speak and how much time to leave between bits of a question is to have an experience as a client yourself.

Eye contact

As when working with spatial processes, make every effort to keep your attention on the metaphor or area of the paper about which you are asking questions rather than making eye contact with your client. This encourages your client to also put his attention on his metaphors rather than on you and your response to them.

So let's start working with metaphors in drawings. I have simplified these Grovian processes a bit to keep them lean and easy to learn and apply.

PROCESS #3 REVISITED: CLEAN LANGUAGE AND METAPHOR MAPS

Designed to:
> Help your client gain greater clarity
> Reveal parts of your client's inner world that are not yet verbalized
> Extend work with a Before Our Session sheet
> Be easily inserted into another Clean process when an appropriate moment presents itself

Useful for:
> Exploring feelings and desires
> Slowing a client down to take more time to notice what there is to notice
> Working with trauma survivors who can use some distance from a difficult subject
> Producing a tangible record of what's been worked on that clients can return to
> End a session

Time to allot: 10–20 minutes

Materials needed:
> Paper for drawing (Copy paper: letter or business size is easy to purchase, store, and carry around. At times, you may prefer to offer a larger size like flip chart paper or a butcher roll.)
> Markers
> Firm drawing surface
> Before Our Session sheet

The Clean Language and Metaphor Map process

I first introduced the use of a drawing to elicit and explore metaphors with Clean Language and the Before Our Session sheet (see page 35) as a way to kick-start a session. Now I am going to expand on how you can work with the Before Our Session sheet drawing so that it can become a larger part of the work you do in a session.

Let's review some Clean questions and a directive we have already covered. The first two are prompts to aid the client in identifying his wants.

> **"And what would you like to have happen?"**

> **"And write or draw what you would like to have happen...or to know more about."**

The second two are used to develop more information about both what the client says and writes and/or draws. Hence, they are known as *developing questions*.

(Where [x] is a word/phrase the client uses)

> **"And is there anything else...about that [x]?"**

> **"And what kind of [x]...is that [x]?"**

With this section's extended Clean Language and Metaphor Map process, you encourage your client to *add to his drawing as new information emerges*. As he describes new elements, you continue to ask the two developing CLQs about the new images *and* about words or phrases he uses in his answers that may not appear on the page (or not yet, at any rate).

Think of it as creating the conditions for emergence: your goal is to help your client collect lots and lots of bits of related information.

To help you help your client evolve his metaphor map, I am going to give you a few more Clean Language questions/directives to use.

The evolving metaphor landscape

As your client talks at length about his drawing, he is likely to describe more metaphors or details about his existing metaphors, and guiding him to find out more about them with the CLQs above is a good facilitation strategy. Particularly important is having your client *locate* the position of an object/figure on his metaphor map because something significant about its relationship to what else is there may be revealed. Realizing, for example, that something the client wants is "within arm's reach" is quite different from discovering that it is "far away" or "out of sight." Using a drawing helps bring such conditions into sharp focus for a client.

When your client mentions a new object, person, or place, repeat his words, and gesturing to his drawing, ask:

> **"And [x]."**

> **"And that would look like what?"**
> or
> **"And [x]."**

> **"And where is that [x]?"**

Notice these phrases are short and simple. Don't elaborate; don't say "Why don't you add that to your drawing?" or "Where would that be if you added that to your picture?" The chattier you get and the more words you use, the more you give your client to process cognitively. You distract him from his focus on his "stuff" and his own mind/body experience of it.

Asking for a new metaphor

At any point in a session your client may talk about a concept, feeling, or state of being, like confidence or love. If it is a *resource* for the client, it will be helpful to find his metaphor for it. Having a vivid way of reconnecting with an embodied sense of a resourceful feeling can provide a client support, motivation, comfort…whatever its value to him might be. If your client finds his internal metaphor for this feeling, he will be better able to connect with it again when he needs it.

The Clean Language prompt to get something conceptual "into metaphor" is:

> **"And [client's word/phrase]."**

> **"And that's [client's word/phrase]…like…what?"**

Note again the dots…for pauses. This question should sound like an invocation, an invitation for something more than added description. Intoning this metaphor-seeking CLQ at a slow, rhythmic pace helps achieve this effect.

Example: Eve

Eve has recently been promoted to her first management position. Having worked with Clean Language before, she has returned to see me, excited to develop a metaphor for the kind of leader she wants to be. We chat for several minutes while she catches me up on her new position.

Eve has brought her Before Our Session sheet with only the top portion filled out; she's made no drawing. This is not particularly unusual. Some clients are more verbally and cognitively oriented, and they do not always take you up on the invitation to draw. Eve has come to me saying she wants to work in metaphor. I just have to pick it up from there.

Under "**And what would you like to have happen?**" Eve has written:

> *I want to be inspiring to others.*

Facilitator: **And what kind of** inspiring **is that** inspiring**?**

Eve: *Like I light up a room!*

Facilitator: **And that would look like what** (gesturing to the paper and markers)**?**

Eve: *A halogen lightbulb.*

Eve draws a long, thin lightbulb, taking time to put detailed marks of some kind on each end.

The unnamed

You have a special challenge when working with a client's drawing, as there may be something on the page—a symbol or a color, for example—that the client adds but does not name. Do not label it yourself! There is no official CLQ for this, so you can create one. But keep it short, simple, and clean. Don't get chatty. For example, I might just gesture toward the added element in the drawing, look expectant, and say,

> "**And what's there…?**" (gesturing to an object, line, etc.)

> or

> "**And is there anything else about…*that*?**" (gesturing to an object, line, etc.)

What if you do that once or twice, and your client does not talk about what you want to call his attention to? Well, that is a good reminder that while that is where *your* attention went, your client's did not. So be it. Stay Clean! Move on to something else.

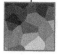

Example: Eve (continued)

Facilitator: **And a** halogen lightbulb. **And what's there?** (gesturing to the ends)

Eve: *Oh, that's important. That's where the connection is made. Without a good connection, there is no light. Others won't see it.*

Anytime a client mentions that something is important, I make a point of asking at least one additional question about it. If the client has found it worthy of singling it out as significant, then it will likely be helpful for her to know more about it.

Facilitator: **And** where the connection is made. **And what kind of** connection **is that** good connection**?**

Eve: *It has to be clean.*

Without my prompt, Eve draws over some lines on each end, making them a bit darker and clearer. Then to the left side, she adds a roundish shape of tiny squiggles.

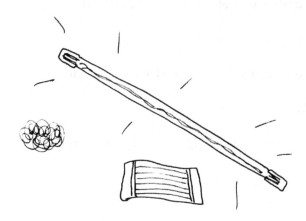

Facilitator: **And what's that?** (gesturing to the roundish shape)

Eve: *This piece of very fine steel wool is to clean the connections with.*

Facilitator: **And** piece of fine steel wool to clean connections with. **And is there anything else about that** clean**?**

Eve: *Yes, I need a cloth to clean fingerprints. The oils from your fingers can be dangerous on halogen bulbs.*

Facilitator: **And that would look like what?**

Eve draws a square next to the bulb and then adds what look like little rays of light coming from the bulb. She says nothing, however.

Facilitator: **And is there anything else about…*that*?** (gesturing to what looks like rays)

Eve: *No. I have what I need to keep the ends clean, and I can light up a room. Everyone sees it now!*

FAQs | *Frequently Asked Questions*

What should I ask questions about?

Simply put: ask about the things the client wants, not about his problems. I know; that's not easy! We are drawn to problems like moths to a flame. We are taught to problem *solve* by examining a problem, dissecting it, and addressing the faults. But what if you were to focus your client's attention instead on getting really familiar with what it is he *wants* first? What a client often discovers is that what he thought was the problem turns out not to be as relevant as he had thought. He may find that what is needed to manifest his want requires a different path altogether. And, not incidentally, getting a clear picture of his goal or intention not only provides new insights; it likely excites and motivates him, putting some new energy behind taking the steps he needs to take. If the problem still intrudes, your client will at least be facing it newly prepared and energized.

What if my client doesn't do a "what I'd like to have happen" drawing? What if despite the instructions, he draws a problem?

Sometimes a client will do this; he will depict the problem state he is in. Perhaps that is all he knows right now. Or he may never have considered what he actually wants, or it is too unclear to even be depicted. It could be that he is simply so focused on his problem that he ignores your question. Whatever the reason, it's okay. He is showing you where his understanding and attention are in the moment.

Get him to describe what he has drawn. Listen attentively, nod sagely, repeat some of his exact words to acknowledge them, and then repeat the starting question, "And what would you *like* to have happen?" If he goes back to talking about the problem? Repeat these steps! And keep on going back to the first question as often as necessary. You might offer a blank piece of paper to him as you ask, not so subtly suggesting that he start a new drawing. You could even say something more conversational (but still Clean of content!) like "And what would it look like if it were what you would *like* to have happen?" Or use James Lawley's go-to: "And when that's what you *don't* want, what would you *like* to have happen?" As soon as your client says or draws anything about what he actually wants, start asking the other CLQs about his words about that.

Suffice it to say that it is not possible in the context of this book on lean Clean processes to go through what to do with every situation that can arise. To learn to work at greater depth and complexity with metaphors, I again refer you to my two workbooks on Grove's Clean Language and its strategic application by Lawley and Tompkins, *Symbolic Modeling* (Campbell, 2102, 2013).

Metaphor maps: Before, during, and/or after a session

- You can have your client do a drawing to begin a session as a way to get started and get some material to work with in another way once you put the drawing aside.

This is the Before Our Session sheet process:

- You can invite your client to continue to add to the drawing (or possibly multiple drawings) as he discovers new details or new symbols. Besides the basic Clean Language questions you have already learned and the ones we just added, you can also apply the next two processes we will cover in this section when an appropriate opportunity arises.

- I always have paper and markers on hand in the event that it seems appropriate to invite my client to create a *metaphor map* at the end of a session even if I have used a spatial process.

Coupling spatial processes and drawing

When using the lean Clean processes in this book that involve space and movement, it is possible that your client will stay largely with everyday or literal material, especially if he is working on some work-related, practical issue. In that case, a drawing may seem irrelevant. But often clients will include one or more seemingly significant metaphors. Having them do metaphor maps after their spatial sessions is another way to help them learn more.

So in Jaime's case once the Clean Space session is done, you could invite her to draw the explorer she mentioned. Depending on your time and intent, you can leave it at that, making no comment on it other than to invite her to describe her drawing if she would like. Simply suggest she take it home with her and put it somewhere where she can see it often as inspiration.

If you still have a couple of minutes, you can ask a few Clean Language questions about it to get her started thinking about it, like this…

Example: Jaime (continued)

Let's pick up with Jaime where she left off (see page 76).

Jaime:	*I feel a huge sense of relief, like it's going to be okay. Phew! All I need to know is the next step. Like any explorer worthy of the name!*
Facilitator:	**And** the next step. **And** an explorer worthy of the name. **And would you like to draw a sketch of that?**
Jaime:	*Oh, great!*

I get out paper and markers and set Jaime up at a table. She spends about five minutes eagerly drawing a picture. Her explorer wears a backpack, topped by a bedroll. There are binoculars around her neck and a canteen at her waist. She has on hiking boots. She is climbing up a mountain, and there are more mountains in the distance.

Facilitator: **And what's here?** (gesturing to the whole drawing)

Jaime: *This is me. I am well prepared for a long trip.*

Facilitator: **And what kind of** well-prepared i**s that** well-prepared**?**

Jaime: *I've got supplies in my backpack: food, extra clothes, matches, a poncho in case of rain. Oh, and a compass but no map. No one's been on my journey before me; there is no map.*

Facilitator: **And** a backpack, clothes, matches, poncho, compass. **And is there anything else about that** compass**?**

Jaime: *With my compass, I can set a course and stay on it if I want to.*

Facilitator: **And what kind of** course **is that** course you can set**?**

Jaime: *Oh, I could set it to explore a particular city or country even. Or I could set it to explore a particular career or just any job that comes across my path that is appealing.*

Facilitator: **And that would look like what?**

Jaime sketches a city skyline in one area of the page and rolling hills in another. She draws several paths or roads through each. In the top right corner, she draws a compass, marking N, E, S, and W.

Facilitator: **And** a compass…and set a course. **And** an explorer worthy of the name. **And what kind of** an explorer **is** an explorer worthy of the name**?**

Jaime: *I think it has to do with being willing to go where no man has gone before… and also willing to follow a beaten path if it feels right. An explorer doesn't always have to be in virgin territory. Plenty of explorers in history had locals who guided them and had crew members to help them. You don't have to go solo to be an explorer worthy of the name. This is about exploring what* you *don't know about, pushing beyond* your *boundaries. Or* my *boundaries, in this case.*

Facilitator: **And** help. **And** pushing beyond your boundaries. **And that would look like what?**

Jaime adds several people beside her figure and a group of three people on a city road and another group of three on one of the valley's roads. No doubt more information about them could be fruitful, but as a facilitator, you have to consider how much time you have and make choices about where to direct your client's attention. With just a few minutes left, I notice Jaime has mentioned a feeling, and I ask a question to get her in touch with her embodied sense of her intuition of what's right for her. It is a *resource* I think she will find useful to get more familiar with.

Facilitator: **And** pushing beyond *your* boundaries. **And** willing to go where no man has gone before. **And** willing to follow a beaten path if it feels right. **And** when feels right, **where is that** feels right?

Jaime: *It's in my gut. Right in the center.*

Facilitator: **And what kind of** a feeling **is that** feeling?

Jaime: *It's a knowing.*

Facilitator: **And** right in the middle of your gut. **And** a knowing. **And it's a** knowing… **like…what?**

Jaime: *Like a compass pointing to true north. I just have to check in, and it will point the way.*

Facilitator: **And that would look like what?**

Jaime adds a small version of the compass in the right corner onto her stick figure's midsection. She puts her markers aside, holds her drawing in front of her, and smiles. She's done.

Jaime: *I'm going to put this right over my desk and check it every day!*

Depending on how you want to work, you could end the session here (see Section 6 for Clean Closure suggestions), or you could transition into another Clean process. My intention with this version of Clean Language and Metaphor Maps is to pan the surface for gold nuggets, and I suspect Jaime would tell you she had found some. We end here.

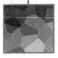

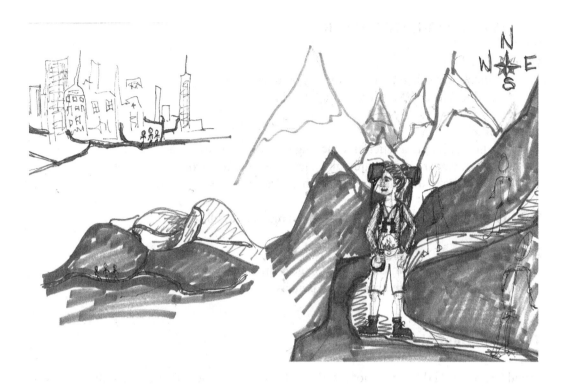

Varying media

Observing clients as they work (1) verbally, (2) moving in space, or (3) drawing, I get the impression (and it is no more than that, as we can't rewind a session and test this) that clients may be accessing different information or be experiencing that information differently by using these different approaches. So I think there is value in having clients who have done a spatial session do a drawing. They use another modality, possibly activating other parts of the brain. Drawing also gives them a way to record what's happened and have something to take home with them. And if they really respond to the drawings, it will give you ideas for using a drawing process in their next session.

In the next two Clean processes we will explore the context of their use with drawings what Grove dubbed Clean Hieroglyphics and Clean Boundaries. Both are Emergent Knowledge processes that elicit bits of information from the subconscious. Both are about *expanding the context* that your client considers so that he might gain a new perspective.

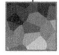

PROCESS #7: CLEAN HIEROGLYPHICS

Designed to:
> Encourage subconscious information to emerge
> Reduce the chance of emotional flooding

Useful for:
> Clients seeking a different coaching or counseling experience
> When you are having difficulty eliciting metaphors from your client
> Clients who include words with their drawing

Time to allot: as few as several minutes or as much as a full session

Materials needed:
> Client's written words on a text page or in a drawing
> A variety of colored markers or pencils

The Clean Hieroglyphics process

David Grove found that it was not just the spoken words a client uses that can open the way for deeper subconscious information to emerge. The way a client writes them down can too. He developed a Clean process he called Clean Hieroglyphics to encourage exploration of written words.

Hieroglyphics refers, of course, to an alphabet used in ancient Egypt in which symbols stood for particular words or sounds. There is something about their pictorial qualities that still seems to appeal to the popular imagination. Why else do so many of us instantly recognize hieroglyphs when few would recognize another ancient script, cuneiform, for example? Perhaps it is their individuality and suggestive wavy lines or their nature and animal forms that invite us to make our own meaning of them. How fitting, then, for Grove to call this exploration of a client's written letters and words Clean Hieroglyphics (or Clean Hiero, as it is referred to for short), for the process is about inviting your client to discover hidden meanings by asking a series of questions that draw his attention to the letters and words he has written, both the lines and the spaces between them. You will notice, like with other Clean questions, they are broad and unspecific.

When a direct approach might be too harsh, threatening, shaming, frightening, or simply mysteriously unhelpful, this more roundabout approach to an issue equips you with a way to structure an exploration for your client that lets him gently discover for himself, at his own pace and in his own order, what it is he is ready to discover.

Evoking your client's metaphor can take him a step closer to the visceral experience of an issue, idea, or event. Asking questions about a representation he makes of his description of it means you are encouraging him to take a step back, to disengage, to make it more abstract. Grove's goal was to take the client "out of the problem space," with its potential emotional intensity and old patterns.

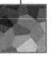

Whether your client zooms in to embody his experience or zooms out to achieve a more distant perspective, it is likely to be different from where he usually consciously experiences his thoughts, feelings, and beliefs about his issue, and thus he may find new information.

You can slip Clean Hiero questions in during any session to briefly explore a written word or phrase, in which case you would spend just a few minutes asking a set of about six questions and then move on. Or if there is lots of written material, you can make Clean Hiero questions the major focus of your session and really give your client time to explore many of the letters and words and their spatial relationships in detail. If your client seems to be getting good information by doing it, why not?

You can use Clean Hiero in response to your client's written words for his want or use this technique when the client includes or adds written words to his metaphor map.

The Clean Hieroglyphics script

Asked about written words on a starting paper or metaphor map:

Step #1: Gathering information (gesturing to paper when asking):

"And what do you notice…about the letters…or words?"

"And what do you notice…about the spaces between the letters…or words?"

"And what do you notice…about the placement of the letters…or words?"

If the client needs a prompt to write or draw the new information on the page, you can either just gesture toward the page or say,

"And that would look like what?"

Stay with any one letter or space or even area of the page too long, and you may get more deeply involved with the emotions and underlying issues involved. If that is not your intention, move on. If you decide to keep on with Clean Hiero, you can use these questions to encourage still more information to emerge. Gesture to what you are referring to when you ask:

"And is there anything else about that letter/word/space/placement?" (when client has singled out one to talk about)

"And what do you notice about any other letters…or words…or spaces?"
"And is there anything else you notice…about what's there?"

"And what do those letters or words or spaces know?"

Or you may ask about a particular letter/word/space if the client has singled it out.

Where [x] is your client's words used in the answer to one of the above questions, you can also ask CLQs for more details about the new information:

"And is there anything else…about that [x]?"

"And what kind of [x]…is that [x]?"

Step #2: Synthesizing

When you are ready to end Clean Hiero, ask this set of questions:

"And what do you know…now?" (gesturing to whole drawing)

"And what do you know now…about [client's original topic/goal]**?"**

"And what difference…does knowing that…make?"

Example: Josh

Josh is a freelance journalist who wants to write a book. He is excited about his topic and the whole idea of writing. He just hasn't gotten moving on it. He has worked with Clean Language before and likes working with his own metaphors, he says, particularly when they surprise him.

Josh: *I want to get on and actually start this new project. I know I can do it. I don't know what's stopping me.*

Facilitator: **And write down or draw what it is you would like to have happen…or to know more about.**

Josh writes the word "KNOW" in capital letters with a blue marker in the center of the page.

Watching Josh take time to write the letters K-N-O-W with such seeming care as to their size and placement on the page and because he has added no other images or symbols, Clean Hiero questions seem like an ideal way to start.

Facilitator: **And what do you notice…about the letters…or word?**

Josh: *Oh, wow. I just noticed that I can add the word* ledge *to* know *and get* knowledge. *Hmm…like I'm on a ledge, on the edge of something new.*

He adds the word "ledge" in smaller letters and the words "of something new" after KNOWl-edge and underlines "edge". Notice Josh did not answer my question about the existing letters or word but added more letters. His attention went elsewhere. Remember: your questions are designed to help your client get more information. If he gets it without your help, that is fine. My next statement acknowledges the new information, and then I repeat the question.

Facilitator: **And** ledge…knowledge. **And is there anything else you notice…about the letters…or words?**

Josh: *It's something about the shape of the N in KNOW. The first line of the N, the one on the left, sort of sweeps, like it has some momentum.*

He writes over the letter in red.

Facilitator: **And what do you notice…about the spaces between the letters…or words…on that paper?**

Josh: *I see there's some space under the word "ledge," beside KNOW, like there's something under it that the letters have to make room for.*

Facilitator: **And what do you know about that** space under "ledge"?

Josh: *I don't really know what this has to do with all this, but this is what comes to me.*

Smiling, he writes the word ZOOM below KNOWledge.

Facilitator: **And what do you notice…about those letters…or that word?**

Josh: *There's momentum in the O's too. They help propel me forward.*

He turns the O's in ZOOM into car wheels and draws a car over them. The top of the car goes into the space under "ledge" and beside KNOW.

Facilitator: **And what do those** O's **know?**

Josh: *They know I can propel myself.*

Facilitator: **And what does the space** under ledge…and beside KNOW **know?**

Josh: *It knows I am the car, and I have the knowledge and the ability to get myself moving.*

Facilitator: **And what do you know…now?**

Josh:	*I realize it's me that gives the wheels their momentum. I can propel myself!*
Facilitator:	**And what do you know now...about** start your new project**?**
Josh:	*I can do it! I have what I need.* (And he adds dots after ZOOM...)
Facilitator:	**And what difference...does knowing all that...make?** (gesturing to whole paper)
Josh:	*I'm glad about that! I didn't know the wheels were there before. And I am the car, and I can steer. I won't just fall off a ledge; I can direct where I'm going and how fast.*

I had thought Josh was finished, and then he adds some more marks to the page. Since we have some time left, I ask a few more questions. My point here is that just because you have come to the end of your list of Clean Hiero questions does not mean you should ignore the answer your client gives. Listen and respond in the moment to what happens. Of course, you could always ask another question...and there has to be a final one at some point. Use your own judgment to determine whether you should keep going, and watch the clock if necessary.

Facilitator:	**And what do** those **know?** (gesturing toward the dots, since Josh has not used a word for them)
Josh:	*They know I have the energy to do it and it can be...it will be...fun.*
Facilitator:	**And are there any other letters...or words...that need to be there?** (gesturing to the whole paper)
Josh:	*Yes. Energy and fun. There will be both!*
Facilitator:	**And that would look like what?**

Josh adds the words "ENergy" in the left bottom corner and "FuN" in the right bottom corner, and writes over the N's in both words in red.

Josh:	*I can't wait to get started!!*

Now he picks up his paper, smiles, and looks up at me. While I would like to ask about energy and fun and the new N's, his behaviors are clear signals that he feels the session is complete. I respect that and end there.

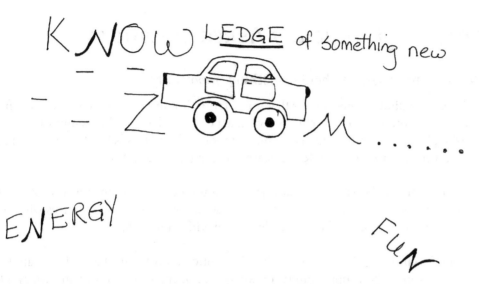

Debriefing

So what just happened? We don't know exactly. Where a different client or even the same client on a different day or with a different topic might have kept talking about practical details about this particular project, this time the client went quickly into metaphor. He seems to have found some energizing inner resource to tap into, and he seems quite pleased about it. Will it make a difference? Only time will tell.

But in case you think what is helpful to a client has to be practical, quantifiable, and found on some expert's checklist or even one you and the client developed in a brainstorming session, let me assure you from experience that those aren't necessarily the things clients are most thrilled to discover or find most useful.

If your client needs that sort of information, well and good. But I find most clients know what they should do; it is just that they are not getting it done. Something else is in the way: they cannot prioritize, they cannot stick to the task list they create for themselves, they make excuses, they lack confidence, they are waiting for the perfect set of circumstances, there is something else they want to be doing more, they cannot let go of something from the past or an old way of doing things...the list goes on. To move to action, it helps if you, the helping professional, use a process that:

- Slows them down and gives them the time and space to stay with one thing long enough to think more deeply about it
- Loosens up the status quo and offers new possibilities
- Empowers them to determine their own solutions
- Helps them access what is presently just out of their conscious awareness
- Helps them find and/or strengthen an inner resource

For the coaching client, often this is enough. For the therapy client, it can be an important step that reveals a hidden spoiler of change and sometimes removes it.

| FAQs | *Frequently Asked Questions* |

What if I miss asking about something important?

"And what kind of important is that important?" Important to whom? If you are using any words other than your client's own exact ones to identify what is important (for example, he says something like "This is important" or "This is what it gets down to"), then you are to a greater or lesser degree, making an assumption.

Your client may provide other cues as to what might be important besides coming right out and labeling it. Listen for words he repeats several times or emphasizes with his voice or with a gesture. Or he may describe it with a metaphor.

And if your question directs your client's attention away from what is significant for him? If you keep the opportunity for emergence open, what is important will eventually come back into your client's awareness, and he will mention it again.

That said, I appreciate your concern. But there is never enough time for a client to attend to everything he could usefully explore. So relax. You cannot know for certain what is going to prove to be most important for your client's healing, growth, or success right now. Getting comfortable with not knowing is something every Clean facilitator adjusts to.

I believe clients are the experts on themselves: they have within more knowledge than we as facilitators could ever surmise. What we can do is help them find that information when it is held subconsciously. We open the conduit and keep the information flowing; determining what knowledge is important and relevant is our client's job.

Should I point out something obvious in my client's writing if he misses it?

What you think is obvious may be incorrect, irrelevant, or less relevant than something else. Stay Clean! Trust the client. Or perhaps, more accurately, I should say, trust the client's subconscious.

Do I have to use all the questions in order?

Your first time through should be a practice session with a friend or colleague, and I suggest you try using all the questions. You can jump about, checking off the ones you have used until they are all checked, or if that is confusing, just go in order. Your intention with the practice should be to get familiar with the questions and asking them smoothly. Since practice is not about giving your "client" the best possible helping or healing experience, find a study buddy. And ideally, have him read the questions for you so you can have an experience as a client too. Once you have a feel for all of the questions, you can work with clients and choose those questions that best fit the logic of the information that emerges. It will not take more than a round or two for you to get comfortable.

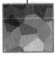

Is Clean Hiero anything like handwriting analysis?

Handwriting analysis works from the premise that your client's subconscious reveals itself in the letters, words, and spaces he writes and they can be deciphered without input from the client. Such analysis is a top-down approach, where theories have been construed about the meaning of writing characteristics and a client's sample ticks off certain pre-determined boxes.

While it is certainly possible that letters, spaces, underlining, capitalizing, punctuation, or even misspelled words may hold meaning, Grovian theory holds that these meanings are individual for the client and that their real usefulness is as a means to help the client better know his inner self. Thus used, they are a tool for bottom-up development.

I suggest another way to consider what is happening is this: by asking Clean questions that offer a client an invitation to make meaning, you provide a way for the subconscious to reveal itself, which it happily takes you up on. I can think of lots of examples of clients making meaning of other things they notice: patterns in a rug, objects in the room, the sound of a plane, or the shape of clouds passing by. I think it most likely that clients are projecting information about their internal systems onto what is handy in the moment, be it their own writing or a nearby object.

As a self-admitted geek about such "Which comes first?" questions, I love thinking about this sort of thing. But when you get right down to it, does it really matter? Whether the subconscious's knowing is revealed on the paper as words are being written or the subconscious takes the invitation to make meaning of what is there to explore and explain itself, or both, the key question is, does asking Clean Hiero questions provide the client with useful information? To which I say, yes, it does.

PROCESS #8: CLEAN BOUNDARIES

Designed to:
> Explore drawn/physicalized lines or symbols that suggest a boundary
> Be used with verbally described or physicalized boundaries

Useful for:
> Identifying an issue's larger context
> Rescaling the significance of an issue

Time to allot: as little as several minutes or can extend to a full session

Materials needed:
> A client's drawing
> A variety of colored markers or pencils
> Extra paper and tape

The Clean Boundaries process

Clean Boundaries is essentially about expanding a client's perspective on an issue. As with all Clean techniques, there is no intent to make anything happen, but what frequently does happen is that the issue is rescaled. That is, seen in a larger context, its significance for the client shifts in a way that is more proportionate to its actual role in his life. That which seemed overwhelming or all encompassing begins to seem like a stage in one's life that can be gotten through or like a manageable issue. Or for a person who feels sad about a given situation or event, he can begin to see it as one part of a larger whole with other parts that are not sad. And so on.

Important: Unique among the processes in this book, this one does not begin with your prompt. This is one that you choose *in response to* what your client writes or draws.

Clean Boundaries can be used with a client's written statement, as with Clean Hiero. Instead of asking about the letters, words, and spaces between them, you will be asking about the space around those words. This may be your plan from the start. Or you could be doing a Clean Hiero series of questions, and your client spontaneously mentions something about the space around his words and adds a line or frame; you pick it up from there, inserting a set of Clean Boundaries questions. It is great to have the two techniques at the ready!

Clients may also draw symbols or metaphors on their metaphor maps that include some kind of a boundary. A path will only be so wide, its edges establishing boundaries on either side. A field, a fence, a gate, a cliff all suggest the client has noticed a boundary. There is some sort of "this side/that side," "inside/outside," or "above/below" to be explored. Ask some Clean questions, and your client may find the two are only subtly different or they may mark the shift from one world to another.

Clean Boundaries is about exploring those boundaries, about extending a client's attention to the spaces beyond his currently perceived boundary.[7] New information can emerge and new perspectives achieved that can bring about dramatic shifts for a client.

Facilitation tips

The same facilitating techniques apply that you use in working with drawing and Clean Language and Metaphor Maps (see pages 81–82). Remember to be attentive to:

- How you pace your questions
- Where you look—at the drawing
- Not touching your client's drawing when he is actively engaged with it

Clean Boundaries script

I have taken some liberties with the wording of these phrases to keep them lean and consistent when possible with phrasing from other processes in this book. There is some wiggle room to vary word selection with Grove's later Clean processes, which he had not vetted as much as his earlier Clean Language phrasing. He experimented and played with the exact wording of his CLQs, sometimes for years, trying to determine which were most helpful to his clients' exploration. We can use small variations and still be true to Grove's work.

Let's assume for our purposes here that your client depicts a boundary at the very start of the session on his Before Our Session sheet so you choose to begin with Clean Boundaries. Or perhaps you have completed a round of Clean Hiero questions about a written statement, and the client has drawn a boundary of some sort and you want to expand on that in a different way.

Step #1: Setting up

Client produces a *drawn or written* statement related to a want that has a boundary or border of some sort.

1. Develop some information about what's delineated by the boundary. It might be words in a box or that have been underlined, or it could be objects for example.

    "And what's that?" (gesturing to objects, shapes, etc.)

    "And is there anything else…about that?" (gesturing to words or objects)

2. Develop some information about the boundary. If the client has not mentioned it yet, ask:

    "And what's that?" (gesturing to boundary demarcation)

    "And is there anything else…about that?" (gesturing to boundary or call by name)

Step #2: Gathering information

Repeat this next set of questions until about *six spaces and boundaries* in all have been explored.

> About spaces:
> 1. **"And what kind of space…is beyond that boundary?"**
> 2. **"And where does that space go?"**
>
> About boundaries:
> 3. **"And what kind of boundary…does that space have?"**

Be sure you give your client time to answer one question before asking the next. Don't rush! If your client mentions some new information that sounds visual, you can add:

"And that would look like what?"

Options

Occasionally, you could ask:

"And is there anything else about there/that?" (gesturing to a space or boundary)

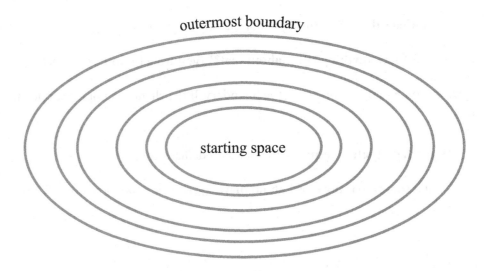

outermost boundary

starting space

To conceive of this process metaphorically, an innermost circle will be established by your first round of questions. Your next round of questions will establish a second circle and so on. Do this until you have six circles, assuming you have enough time and that your client continues to discover new information.

Warning: don't be misled by the graphic above. There is no rule that says the spaces must be geometrically perfect or the same distance apart or in any other way be regular.

Your client may want to rewrite or redraw his picture or attach other pieces of paper as his landscape expands. Be sure you have more paper and tape if your client wants to connect multiple pieces. It is all part of the rescaling that is going on.

Step #3: Reversing direction

Once your client has gone out as many spaces as you determine to go out, up to about six, go back in reverse order, checking to determine what is known now. In each case, gesture toward the boundary or area you are asking about.

> **"And what does that boundary know?"**

> **"And what does that space know?"**

Add **"And that would look like what?"** when client mentions additional information on images.

Continue on until you reach the original written words or objects, and ask:

> **"And what does that** [word/object] **know?"**

Options

Occasionally, you could ask:

> **"And is there anything else that space knows?"**

> **"And is there anything else that boundary knows?"**

Step #4: Synthesizing

End with these Clean questions:

> **"And what do you know…now?"**

> **"And what do you know now…about** [original topic/goal]**?"**

> **"And what difference…does knowing that…make?"**

But as with other processes, do not use these every time or too often. Keep your client moving!

Example

If Clean Boundaries sounds a bit complicated to facilitate, trust me. When your client's drawing is in front of you, it is quite easy to keep track of identifying new spaces and boundaries and then revisiting them in reverse.

There are extensive examples of Clean Boundaries in a couple's session starting on page 160. Because of its length with both the husband's and wife's experiences, I will not put yet another example here. I think you will find it intriguing in the context of their full session.

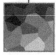

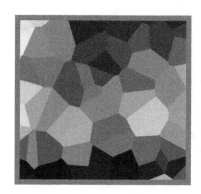

Making a Plan

I began this book talking about some of the concepts and intentions underlying David Grove's processes, including how people change. Essentially, Grove was looking to help the client gather information that will spark a new, emergent organization of his mind/body system if it is needed.

That said, Grove did not maintain that you need to leave everything to spontaneous emergence alone. Some Clean questions and processes are designed to help your client cement change, act on it, and prevent relapse. There are:

- CLQs that move time forward to take the client further into his new reality so he can get comfortable with it. This way he is less likely to slip back into the old, familiar way (Campbell, 2012).

- CLQs that encourage unresolved problems to reveal themselves, the sometimes hidden causes of relapse (Campbell, 2013).

- CLQs that ask the client to put his attention on the entirety of the new whole, reinforcing the new, transformed order.

- Clean processes to help a client develop a list of concrete actions.

It is these last two that we will focus on in this section.

Let's begin by reviewing some CLQs you have already learned from the perspective of moving the client from examining himself to taking his newfound knowledge, awareness, feelings, perspective, ideas, etc., out into the world.

SYNTHESIZING

Some Clean questions ask the client to reflect on what he has experienced and learned as a whole. In addition to inviting new awareness and structuring, the questions are meant to solidify and reinforce any changes. And they are the first steps toward bringing changes from his inner life into his active, external life. I've found these to be powerful questions, and I often ask one or both at the end of any of the extensive Clean processes. They should be familiar to you by now.

"And when all that,…what do you know…now?"

"And what do you know now…about [goal/topic of inquiry]**?"**

"And what difference…does knowing all that…make?"

Let's take a moment to reflect on what the second question encourages, as it is distinctly different than any other CLQ you have learned. The question invites your client to:

- **Acknowledge:** He slows down and appreciates that he really has found something of value. Sometimes he gives himself credit for something important, or he recognizes something is truly giving him relief. He may have found a key piece to a puzzle that has been bothering him for some time. This question gives him time to acknowledge and relish whatever it is.

- **Assess:** If the last "And what do you know now?" question is the apex of his experience, if he has been panning away and this is his gold, this second question gently asks him to go still one step further. It asks for a cognitive assessment of the experience, inviting him to move from engaging with his psychoactive space into conscious processing. It nudges him to go beyond an awareness of his experience and insights to make meaning of them.

- **Generalize:** He may realize that his insight pertains not just to his topic for the day but more broadly in his life as he steps back to consider the whole of his experience.

- **Ground:** It helps to ground him back in "ordinary" time and space.

- **Segue:** If you choose to use this question to end one of the Clean processes we have covered so far, it makes a fine transition into our next lean processes, Clean Action and Clean Action Space, that invite your client to make specific plans to apply what he has learned.

Even if you are not using a Clean process, these are great questions to use with your clients as you come to the end of your sessions.

TAKING ACTION

Researchers Rodgers, Milkman, John, and Norton determined that making a plan significantly increases the likelihood that subjects will act on their intentions. *Telling* someone else about one's intentions increases that likelihood still further. Interestingly, this was particularly true for subjects who were the most enthusiastic. It seemed they thought their fervor would carry them through without the need for a plan, but that did not turn out to be the case.[8]

David Grove developed Clean Action and Clean Action Space for the times it is appropriate to help a client create a clear game plan for follow-up actions. The processes are particularly useful for coaches who are outcome oriented, but increasingly therapists include solution-oriented behavioral goals as part of their therapy as well.

So what signals indicate an appropriate time?

A client may use words to describe wanting or needing to take *actions* or *steps, make plans* or a *to-do list.*

He may be vaguer: *"I don't know how to start"* or *"I'm not sure what to do first"* or *"I'm good with the big picture, but not with details."* These phrases suggest he would benefit from making a list of details or steps to take. But don't decide for him; simply ask, for example,

> **"And when** you not sure what to do first**, what would you like to have happen?"**

If your client says he wants to make a plan or list, here are two clean ways to do that. Because they use Clean Language wording for the questions and directives, they combine very nicely with the other Clean processes.

Why use a Clean process to get a list of actions?

Can't you simply get your client to list specific actions in a more conversational way? You can, to be sure. Many coaching models detail ways to do just that. But consider the advantages of using Clean questions.

- You may slip into being *un-Clean* if you do not use Grove's Clean questions and a structure. Especially when it comes to making plans, you may be tempted to offer well-intentioned suggestions and advice. But your client may have already tried what you suggest, and then he will end up wasting his time and attention to explain to you what was not successful. Or he may assume your suggestions will not work, or he is not enthusiastic about trying them but will not speak up. Why not let your client discover his solutions for himself? Hold the space. Give him uninterrupted time and attention. Empower him to know and rely on himself.

- Clean questions foster a different way of listening to oneself and one's words than normal conversation does. Grove's unusual question structure and very simple, sparse words will continue to invite your client to search for answers from his deeper places of knowing even though he is thinking more about the everyday world of actions.

- Clean Action Space offers the additional advantage of working in the client's psychoactive space, a decidedly different experience than typical cognitive methods for creating lists.

You may, indeed, have some information or advice that your client will find useful in making plans, and you may choose to make space for that in your time together. But beware of *assuming* what it is your client needs based on your professional judgment and experience with clients *in general* as opposed to what your client has made very clear is *his* need. Having the opportunity to hear what your client comes up with for actions and steps will reveal a lot.

If you are surprised by his answers, that's revealing, too. When I am surprised, it lets me know I probably made inaccurate assumptions. Maybe they were about what a client knows already or needs first or what he is ready for.

In any case, hold back on launching into information or advice giving as long as you can. Hear your client out until he has no more to add before making any contributions of your own. You will be much more likely to be successful at meeting him exactly where he is with exactly what information he needs.

PROCESS #9: CLEAN ACTION

Designed to: Specify active steps that move the client from introspection to action

Useful for:
> Measuring progress
> Encouraging a sense of accountability
> Sustaining motivation
> Reinforcing the message that the client is the expert on himself

Time to allot: varies from 10 minutes to the entire session

Materials needed: Notepad for recording results

The Clean Action process

You can use these Clean questions to help your client get really specific about how he will carry his new awareness or understanding into his life. The goal is to come up with executable actions your client can and will take. As with any Clean process, the client is the one who is wholly responsible for coming up with the plan's contents.

Your role is to hold the time and space for him to do it, keeping him focused on identifying specific and doable actions.

Note taking

Before you begin Clean Action with your client, set him up with paper and pen. He will need to keep track of the items in his plan. Physically engaging in the act of writing:

- Signals to him that he is taking responsibility for these actions.
- Slows him down. Who knows what will emerge with more time and attention?
- May increase his commitment to do what he says he wants to do.

Of course, if your client's age or physical health limits his ability to take notes, you may offer to help. Be sure you are recording his act words! He could also make an audio recording of the session for himself.

Clean Action script

Step #1: Establishing a goal [x]

> **"And what you would like to have happen?"**

If the answer is a goal that can be met with actions and you are at this planning stage with your client, you can choose Clean Action.

Step #2: Gathering information

First action:

> **"And what's an action you know you can do...to [x]?"**
>
> **"And how will you do that?"** (repeat until the action is quite specific)
>
> **"And when will you do that?"** (repeat until the answer is specific)

Then ask for about five more actions:

> **"And what's another action you know you can do...to [x]?"**
>
> **"And how will you do that?"** (repeat until the action is quite specific)
>
> **"And when will you do that?"** (repeat until the answer is specific)

Specific *action* means it should be an observable behavior. *Hows* could include where, how long, with whom, with what materials, and so on. A specific *when* is not "soon" but "next Wednesday, after work."

Step #3: Synthesizing

> **"And what do you know...now?"**
>
> **"And what difference...does knowing that...make?"**

Options

1. **Ask for more specifics.**

   "And is there anything else about that action you know you can do...to [x]?"

   "And is there anything else about how/when you will do that?"

2. **Come back for the *hows* and *whens*.** You have the option of getting a list of the actions first and going back to ask *how* and *when* for each one once the list is complete. Personally, I prefer getting a list first because my client can get caught up in a problem with the execution of one action and get sidetracked, potentially running out of time to get back to completing that list. And it is likely he will have a few items that seem manageable, even easy, and knowing this can help motivate or sustain a client who has found one of his items is more challenging. You may prefer getting all the information about an item at once. Or you may notice your client has a preference.

Example

Though Clean Action is a verbal process and the next one, Clean Action Space, is spatial and thus can feel quite different to a client, they are so similar to one another in terms of the script that I will let one example in this section suffice for them both. I am confident you can adjust to their differences. For a few Clean Action questions used in a session, read Matt's example (see page 182).

PROCESS #10: CLEAN ACTION SPACE

Designed to: Specify active steps that move your client from introspection to action

Useful for:
> Measuring progress
> Encouraging a sense of accountability
> Sustaining motivation
> Reinforcing the message that the client is the expert on himself

Time to allot: 15–45 minutes

Materials needed: Notepad for recording results

The Clean Action Space process

In Clean Action Space your client moves around to various spaces, discovering what he knows from those locations about what actions he wants to take to reach his goal. The Clean questions are worded slightly differently than in Clean Action, accordingly.

Now, you could conduct a Clean Space session with the topic of inquiry being an action the client wants to take and very cleanly and open-endedly invite your client to locate spaces to find out more about that goal. But your client may or may not get a list of doable actions. Clean Action Space is for the times your client has said he wants to create a list or plan. It is more directive than Clean Space.

Note taking

Before you begin, discuss with your client who will take notes for your client to have to take with him. Because this process involves moving about, it may end up being you. If you feel strongly about the advantages of having your client do the writing himself for kinesthetic reinforcement, you could have him make a copy of your notes to take with him. Just be sure you get his exact words. Or let him record this session for himself if the microphone can handle the moving about.

Clean Action Space script

Step #1: Establishing a goal [x]

> **"And draw or write what you would like to have happen."** (gesturing to the paper and markers)

or

> **"And choose an object to represent what you would like to have happen."**

If the answer is a goal that can be met by taking actions and you are at this planning stage with your client, you can choose Clean Action Space.

Step #2: Setting Up

> **"And put that** (gesturing to paper/object) **where it seems...right."** (gesture around the room)

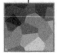

Step #3: Gathering information

First action:

>"And find a space that knows about an action you can to do…to [x]."

>"And from there…what do you know you can do…to [x]?" (gesture to paper/object)

>"And how will you do that?" (repeat until the action is quite specific)

>"And when will you do that?" (repeat until the answer is specific)

Ask for about five more actions:

>"And find a space that knows about another action you can do…to [x]."

>"And from there…what do you know you can do…to [x]?" (gesture to paper/object)

>"And how will you do that?" (repeat until the action is quite specific)

>"And when will you do that?" (repeat until the answer is specific)

Step #4: Synthesizing

>"And find a space…that knows about all this." (gesturing to all the spaces)

>"And from there…what do you know…now?"

>"And what difference…does knowing that…make?"

Option

>"And is there anything else from there…you know you can do…to [x]?"

>"And is there anything else about how/when you will do that?"

Ending

Determine for yourself how you would like to end the session. You may offer the notes you've taken to your client to keep and to revise. Keep a copy yourself so you will have it to refer to at your next session when you check in with your client to see what he has accomplished. Or your client could make a copy for himself; this gives him an opportunity to modify it.

Example: Jaime (continued)

Remember Jaime, the college art major? (see pages 89–91) We left off with her after using a Clean Language and Metaphor Map process. But what if I had taken a different approach? What if when Jaime said "All I need to know is the next step," I had taken that as a cue to do a Clean Action Space session to develop a list of actions to take. I would have guided her in a very different direction and gotten a very different kind of information. I think you will find the comparison useful.

So here is how Jaime's Clean Action Space session might have gone. You will notice that I mostly stick to the script, but sometimes another Clean Language question seems called for. I will also use the option to get a list of actions first and then go back to get the *how's* and *when's*. Let's rewind the Metaphor Map session and go back to where it started.

Jaime: *I feel a sense of relief, like it's going to be okay. Phew! All I need to know is the next step. Like any explorer worthy of the name!*

Facilitator: **And all you need to know is the next step. And write or draw that.** (gesturing to post-its and markers)

Jaime writes "Next step" on the post-it.

Facilitator: **And put that where it seems…right.**

Jaime pulls the coffee table in to the center of the open space in the room and puts the post-it on it.

Facilitator: **And find a space that knows about an action you can do…to** know the next step. (gesturing to the post-it)

Jaime wanders around a bit until settling into a space near the window.

Facilitator: **And from there…what do you know you can do…to** know the next step? (gesturing to the post-it)

Jaime: *I can broaden my thinking, my search for a job. I was just thinking painting and set design, but I'm excited now to explore other options. I want to start exploring new possibilities.*

It's a fine visionary answer that may inspire Jaime, but there are actions specified. I repeat the question, adding a few of her new words to acknowledge them.

Facilitator: **And from there…what do you know you can do…to** start exploring new possibilities and know the next step? (gesturing to the post-it)

Jaime: *I could go back to the career counseling office and talk with Shelley. She was helpful before, and now I can go with a different set of questions.*

It seems logical to encourage Jaime to be more specific here before moving on.

Facilitator: **And what** questions **could those** questions **be?**

Jaime: *Like get some ideas about other careers that don't involve fine arts directly. Things that are creative and hands on 'cause I really like that. But I don't know…other things. That's what I'll get Shelley to help me figure out: how to search for creative ideas and options on the Internet.*

Facilitator: **And how will you** talk with Shelley?

Jaime: *Oh, I'll just stop by the career counseling office. No, better yet, I'll call first and see what days she's there and make an appointment with her.*

Facilitator: **And when will you** talk with Shelley?

Jaime: *Oh, I can do that right after we're finished here.*

Facilitator: **And find a space that knows about another action you can do…to** know the next step.

And from there…what do you know you could do to know the next step?

Jaime: *Well, I know I can call two friends who graduated last year who were art majors too. They're living in New York. I'm not sure what they're doing now, but I think it'd be good to talk with them. Maybe they'll have some ideas, know about some people who've tried different things. I might get some ideas from them.*

Facilitator: **And how will you do that?**

Jaime: *I have Eliza's email already. Jack's on Facebook. So I can get both their numbers easily.*

Facilitator: **And when will you** get their numbers?

Jaime: *I can do that right after this too.*

Facilitator:	**And when will you** call them?
Jaime:	*I'll wait until early tonight when they're probably at home. No, wait! I'll wait to call them until after I've talked to Shelley and poked around on the Internet a bit. I might have better questions to ask them if I wait until then.*

I see a potential problem, so I adapt a Clean question to the situation.

Facilitator:	**And how much** poking around **will you** do?
Jaime:	*Oh, I see. Yeah, I could poke around forever, I guess. Okay. Let's say I'll look around until I get three new ideas and then I'll call Eliza and Jack.*
Facilitator:	**And find a space that knows about another action you can do…to** know the next step. **And from there…what do you know you could do to** know the next step**?**
Jaime:	*I'm going to look into possible internships. They might be a better way to explore possibilities I haven't considered before than trying to get a job doing something I've done.*
Facilitator:	**And how will you do that?**
Jaime:	*That one's going to be harder. I can get Shelley to get me started. And maybe my art department profs can make some suggestions. Maybe they'll have some connections. I can check with my advisor.*
Facilitator:	**And** Shelley can get you started. **And** check with your advisor. **And how will you** check with your advisor**?**
Jaime:	*I'll email him and ask him when I can come in to talk with him.*
Facilitator:	**And when will you** email him?
Jaime:	*I'll add it to today's list. These are all short and easy things, these emails.*
Facilitator:	**And find a space that knows about all this.** (gesturing to all the spaces) **And from there…what do you know…now?**
Jaime:	*I know that I'm a lot more relaxed with a plan and specifics. I feel less adrift in the Unknown.*

And she smiles as she gestures to the space where Unknown was in her Clean Space session. She hadn't forgotten!

Facilitator: **And what difference…does knowing that…make?**

Jaime: *It feels good to have things spelled out like this. I love checking off lists! This is good.*

Facilitator: And as you look over your list, **is there anything else** you want to add or delete or change?

Jaime: *No, this is plenty. I feel like it's a good plan.*

What you do next depends to some extent on the contract you have with your client and perhaps a company or organization you work for. But assuming for the moment that the choice is yours alone, resist the urge to give a client like Jaime other suggestions you could think of, tempting as it may be.

She has listed quite a few good ideas on her own, and even if you think some are unlikely to pan out, let her find that out on her own, building her learning and confidence as she goes. She is going to feel a lot more empowered and self-sufficient if she acts on her own ideas and something comes from them than if she acts on yours. Try saving them for next time if they are needed, and stay Clean!

Facilitator: **And would this be a good place to stop for right now?**

Jaime: *Yeah, great!*

Facilitator: Would you like to copy this list down? I like to keep a copy to be sure to have it next time we talk.

Jaime: *Sure. I'd like to put it in my phone, actually.*

Comparing processes

If you have not already done so, go back and reread the Metaphor Map session I did with Jaime (see pages 89–91). Strikingly different from this one, isn't it? As a counselor, I am far more likely to choose the Metaphor Map process for Jaime until she has done the sort of self-exploration the metaphor work elicits. If I were a career counselor, I might feel the Clean Action Space choice to be more appropriate. Your choice of processes will depend on what stage your client is in in his work with you and your contract with him.

FAQs | Frequently Asked Questions

I can see where I could spend a lot of time with a client having him come up with actions. If my client seems to be on a roll, should I just keep asking for more actions?

You could keep asking for more actions until your client runs out of ideas if you have enough time. But you want to be careful not to overwhelm your client with so many actions to take that he can't reasonably accomplish them in the near future. The intent of Clean Action and Clean Action Space is to help your client come up with a specific *doable* list. To keep a client motivated and hopeful, keep the number of actions manageable and help him chunk them down into specific steps.

What if my client leaves out a really obvious, necessary action he needs to be taking? Aren't I taking a risk that he'll think I'm inadequate at helping him or our working together isn't successful once he realizes what needs to be done?

First of all, the action may be obvious to you, but evidently it isn't to him. If and when this action step does become clear to your client, it may seem to him more like a new awareness, or it may come with the realization that it was something he wasn't letting himself acknowledge. In either case, with a Clean process that uses his words and so clearly works from a place of where the client is at the moment, why would that be your fault? If he does blame you, then that is something to explore. If it worries you, just be sure you have set up your contract and the expectations of what you will be providing very clearly.

Your job is to help enable your client to accomplish his ultimate goal. You may see the giant steps he needs to take, and he is only seeing baby steps directly in front of him. Maybe on some level he is aware that one of those steps involves strengthening a resource first—such as building the confidence to take giant steps…a part of his process you may not be privy to. As long as your client is not putting himself or someone else in danger or suggesting something illegal or unethical or that could otherwise lead to a seriously damaging outcome your client is just not seeing, trust his wisdom.

To return to your question, you may feel strongly that a certain action is necessary. And it may well be, but are you sure it is necessary just now? The intent of Clean Action and Clean Action Space is not to uncover and work on accomplishing difficult steps (though they may emerge during the process) but on your client's identifying doable actions. This may require you refrain from pointing out what you think needs to be done to accomplish a goal vs. what your client says he can do.

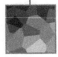

And too—what we are talking about in this book are lean techniques. When things get more complicated and more challenging, other approaches may be called for.

What if my client says there are no actions he wants to take or only comes up with one or two?

That's fine. You ask the questions with sincere curiosity and accept the answers without judgment. Perhaps your client needs time to digest what has emerged for him. If you have used another Clean process before this one, he may have gone to a deeper, more intuitive space within, and getting analytical and practically oriented is not where he wants to go right now. Staying Clean means you do not make assumptions about what your client is ready to do. If he says he is done, then he is done.

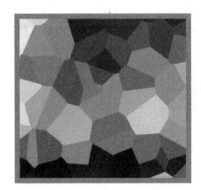

Clean Closures

Your contract with your client, the goal of the session, or the way you work could point to different ways of bringing your session to a close. Some of the processes we have covered that can take up a full session, such as Clean Networks or Clean Space, have endings built right in, and you may be fine stopping your Clean session there. With others, you may feel you need a graceful way to wrap things up. It could seem abrupt and unsatisfactory if you were literally to stop your session with your client's last answer to one of the Clean questions. So how might you close out the session?

First of all, stay Clean. Just because you are no longer using one of the Clean processes doesn't mean it is appropriate to start giving advice or adding your own observations. Give information, perhaps, but not advice, not your take on your client's stuff. Remember, you are not there to fix things for him; you are there to empower him to fix things for himself.

Beware of labeling your client's experience for him. It is easy to unintentionally do you're trying to be empathetic and fall back into old habits.

Examples

"Wow. That was powerful!"
"You had some difficult moments there."
"I sense you are…(fill in the blank)."
"You came up with a really creative solution!"

No matter how what body language you observe or what comments your client makes, be sure to use only his words to describe his experience.

Getting conversational

Here are a few suggestions for helping your client gently get his normal boundaries and way of interacting with others back in place.

1. Say something along the lines of:

    "And take all the time you need over the next days or weeks to… (and here you adjust your wording to what was said in the session).

    …get more familiar with [x]."

    …notice more about [y]."

    …see what happens next."

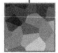

Example

Client: *I feel this connection now between my head and my heart, like a river flowing between them. My head just got in the way before of being clear on what I truly want, but now I know I can trust my answers because my heart is connected to and communicating with my brain.*

Facilitator: **And take all the time you need in the next days and weeks to become more familiar with** that connection between your heart and brain…like a river flowing between them…**and see what happens next when** your heart is connected to and communicating with your brain like that.

I highly recommend you work out a little script for yourself with this sort of ending because it is easy to find yourself sort of blithering away, making it all too easy not to stay Clean!

2. Ask:

"And as we're just about out of time,…is there anything else about all that… for right now?"

This gives your client one last opportunity to finish up. But be careful who you offer this invitation to! If you know your client is one to talk on incessantly, oblivious to the warning that your time is about up, then do not use this choice to close!

You can use this one alone or tack it on at the end of #1.

3. Ask:

"And would this be a good place to stop…for right now?"

The emphasis here on "stop" rather than "anything else" makes it a firmer call to end. (You may have noticed I used this question to end the example session in the last chapter on page 117.)

You can use this one alone or tack it on at the end of #1.

The examples above employ Clean Language's hypnotic syntax and pacing. When you are ready to resume normal conversation, you can:

4. Change your tone and speed up the pace at which you are speaking so that it is more natural. But do not go from 0 to 60! That feels uncomfortably abrupt when you are coming out of trance. Speed up gradually.

5. Look your client in the eye, as in normal conversation. Referring to him by his name is another way of bringing him out of his inner exploration.

6. If you have not already developed a plan using Clean Action or Clean Action Space, you could assign some other sort of homework (like "Draw a *metaphor map* when you get home.")

7. Get practical. It will bring your client back to a more cognitive way of thinking. Looking at the calendar to schedule your next session or dealing with payment will do it.

It is important to get your client grounded again in the everyday world. Doing a Clean process can put your client in a deeply mindful, spacey sort of place, and you want to make sure your client is "back" before going down a flight of stairs or driving a car. I imagine a deep sea diver. You want to bring a client back up to the surface of everyday reality, but do so gradually and gently. Be sure to leave at least five minutes for this.

Ending on a positive note

Not every session is going to end with your client having resolved all his issues, of course. Life isn't always straightforward, and change can be complicated. But you do want to send your client off feeling resourceful.

Recall our definition of resources: anything—an object, a person, a feeling, a skill—whatever it is that an individual identifies as being useful or of value in a particular context. For a client to leave a session feeling resourceful means he feels he has something or someone he can turn to that will help him cope.

Now, you may be thinking that is what you are: a resource to him he can rely on! But do you really want him to rely on you to cope? Do you want to encourage that kind of dependence? Certainly not in the long run. I am not saying your client may not think of you that way, but that doesn't mean you have to encourage it.

Consider something that might have come up in the session that your client identified that is a good resource. Maybe he knows about ways to relax in stressful situations. Maybe he described a feeling of confidence he can call upon when needed. Maybe he identified a place to go when he gets overwhelmed where he can sort things out. Maybe he noted that when he steps away from a heated argument for 20 minutes, he returns better able to resolve a problem in a productive way. A resource can be a place, some self-talk, a friend or family member, an emotion, an action, and so on. The less it is reliant on someone else, the more internalized it is, the better. Then it is always there for your client.

If a Clean session ends on a generally discouraging note, take some time to review the resources your client mentioned and remind him of what he said by saying his words back to him. And notice, I said to refer to a resource *your client mentions*. If, for example, your client never mentioned having a family who loves him, making the assumption that his family is, in fact, loving and is naturally a resource could be a big mistake. Make no assumptions. Stick to your client's words. Stay Clean.

Ideally, the client identifies the resource he singles out as being most helpful now, so be listening for it. Here is an example of how a facilitator might respond to a client's words, reviewing them to encourage him to put his attention on this newfound resource.

Example

Facilitator: **And** you don't know if you can speak your truth to him yet. **And** it's going to take some time to find out. **And** you're okay with that. **And** confidence… an oak tree in your spine, growing bigger bit by bit.

Once you have reviewed a resource, you can use this next activity to help concretize it in your client's mind/body, giving him a strong visual image and ideally a strong visceral experience of it to come back to.

Ending with a metaphor map

If you used a Clean spatial process or if you used a talking process, Clean or otherwise, you can bring that portion of the session to a close by inviting your client to draw, breaking from the question/directive and answer rhythm of the Clean process you want to finish. Be sure to leave time for this; my clients generally take 5 to 10 minutes.

Invitation:

> **And what could that** oak tree growing bit by bit…in your spine…**look like?** (gesturing toward paper and markers)

A more conversational version:

> **And when** confidence **is like an** oak tree growing bit by bit in your spine, **would you like to make a sketch of that?**

When he indicates he has finished drawing, you can invite your client to talk about it as you listen attentively and respond briefly, conversationally, but still Cleanly.

If it seems appropriate, you could encourage your client to take the sketch home and put it somewhere where he can see it: the refrigerator door, a desk drawer (if he wants to keep it private), the bathroom mirror. I find clients appreciate the suggestion that they can use their metaphor maps—and their memories of their embodied experience of their metaphors—to remind and inspire them of what they discovered in their sessions.

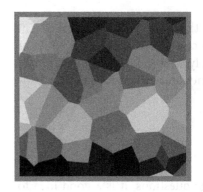

Section Seven

Clean Processes
with Groups

Next we will consider two types of groups you might use Clean processes to facilitate. The first type of group consists of individuals working on their own issues, which may or may not share a common theme. The second type of group is one with an intention to collaborate in some way, whether the members form a couple, a family, a class, a business, or some other sort of team. This section presents a Clean process to use for each of these.

ADAPTING CLEAN PROCESSES TO GROUPS

A number of the processes we have covered so far can be adapted for groups. Each individual can learn something about himself as you offer guiding Clean questions for a number of people at once.

Your Clean script will differ in that rather than referring to the topic or words a single client identifies, you use a general word to refer to something each individual names silently for himself. You may call it "goal" or "topic" or "issue" or simply refer to it as "that." Just let the group members know what word you will be using and encourage them to silently substitute their own words if they want to.

Demonstration

If this is the group's first experience with Clean Language questions, it is a good idea to demonstrate the questions you will ask briefly with a volunteer to be sure everyone understands what to expect and has an opportunity to ask questions without disturbing the group once you begin.

Be sure that participants are clear that they will not speak their answers aloud, as your volunteer may do.

Pacing

I find the greatest challenge when facilitating multiple individuals working spatially or with evolving drawings at the same time is the timing of the questions. Inevitably one person will be looking at me, waiting for me to go on, while another has just seemed to settle in and get started. I suggest letting the group know that you will try to keep a steady pace and that you will tend to give a bit more time rather than less. Encourage those who have "gotten" their answers to ask themselves silently "And is there anything *else* about that?" Those members who feel rushed can take some private time later to reflect further.

After the guided process

You can decide, depending on your context, what you will have participants do with their responses. For example, you may have them divide into groups of two or three and share within the small group. If your entire group has eight or fewer members and you have the time, they might all share with one another.

An issue that I find often arises is how other participants should respond to another's sharing. I suggest you come up with some guidelines beforehand to prepare for this. My own sense is that the surest way to create a safe place for sharing is to encourage people to stay Clean (whether you use this term or not). The listener's role is to be a witness and in some cases, to encourage the sharer's further self-discovery with Clean questions.

The listener's role is not to share his similar experiences, make suggestions, or offer other interpretations. It is not to criticize *nor is it to give praise*. Both are forms of judgment that pull the speaker's attention away from his own experience and toward how others see him. Whether that triggers defensiveness or the desire to please or earn acceptance, it is a distraction at best, and at its worst, it could undermine growth and self-healing.

If the listeners stay Clean, those who share will feel safe from judgment, and participants will learn to listen and respond without introducing their own content, a useful skill for conversing with anyone in any context.

So what can you as the facilitator or the other participants say when it feels right to say *something*? How about "Thank you for sharing," followed by a pause that accords what has been shared some honored space to be held by the group. If you establish this as the go-to response at the outset, it will feel appropriate.

Another possible way to have participants process their experiences once you have finished facilitating is to give them some quiet time for contemplation: to write, draw, or simply sit or walk quietly. I have found 15 minutes to do this when the memory of it is freshest has been deeply appreciated. But this depends on the group, its purpose, and the time available.

So which processes you have learned so far lend themselves to individual work in a group setting? Consider using:

Group Clean Spinning

See script on page 195. Adjusting this to a group is effortless. Just be sure participants are spread out at least an arms-width apart, hopefully further, to allow each person more free visual space around him. Have participants identify what they would "like to have happen or know more about" and get them spinning!

Group Clean Networks

See script on page 196. This process applied to a group is also straightforward. Only for this process, your participants are likely to need more space. That said, in the extreme, you can facilitate this process when each person has no more space than a piece of paper on his lap. He can simply identify his spaces with a marker or by placing a coin or other token. Most people adjust easily to whatever the space parameters are.

Just be sure you are keeping your voice slow, slightly hypnotic and rhythmic, at a pace that invites participants to go inside for their answers. If you speak too quickly, in a clipped, conversational manner, your participants will "stay in their heads," getting information from the same cognitive places they usually go. What a missed opportunity that would be!

Group Clean Action

See script on page 204. If you have been facilitating a group using one of these Clean processes or some other activities and it is time to make some concrete action plans, you can use Clean Action to guide independent planning. Be sure to leave time to have participants share their action plan with at least one other person; remember, research shows people are more likely to follow through on their plans if they have told someone else about them, and group members can serve this purpose.[9] Alternatively, you can have the participants work in pairs, providing them with a facilitator's script and let them guide each other through their planning processes.

Here, in more detail, is how you can repurpose Clean Language and the Before Our Session sheet for a group with individual goals.

PROCESS #11: CLEAN METAPHOR MAPS IN A GROUP SETTING

Designed to:
> Encourage personal development
> Help group members know one another better, understand and appreciate their similarities and differences, priorities, thinking, expectations, etc.

Useful for:
> Group therapy
> Workshop groups
> Families/couples
> Team work groups

Time to allot: depending on the size of the group, 20–60 minutes

Materials: plain paper and markers

Clean Metaphor Maps for individuals in a group setting process

Step #1: Setting up

Have each person complete a Before Our Session sheet (see script on page 194). Be sure you spend a few moments to make it clear that stick-figure drawings are fine; this need not be about being artistic.

Step #2: Gathering new information

Once participants have completed their sheets, let them know you will be asking a series of questions while they look at their drawings and that they will be invited to add to their drawings as new information emerges.

As I mentioned before, the biggest challenge in working with groups like this is pacing your questions. Inevitably, it will be too fast for some and too slow for others. Encourage patience and a willingness to keep open to discovering more answers if they find themselves waiting for the others in the group.

Step #3: Synthesizing

You are familiar with this step by now. This is where participants reflect on the meaning or significance of what they have discovered.

Clean Metaphor Maps for individuals in a group setting script

Step #1 Setting up

Invite participants to complete Before Our Session sheets (see sample on page).

Step #2: Gathering new information

Ask these Clean Language questions, allowing plenty of time between each:

> **"And as you look at what that would look like…, what are you drawn to?"**

> **"And what do you know…about that?"**

> **"And that would look like what?"** (gesturing to draw/write on paper)

"And what else do you know…about that?"

"And that would look like what?" (gesturing to draw/write on paper)

Repeated rounds

Depending on the time available, you can repeat this set of questions up to five more times. For each round, ask:

"And looking at that drawing again,…what are you drawn to?"

"And what do you know…about that?"

"And that would look like what?" (gesturing to draw/write on paper)

"And what else do you know…about that?"

"And that would look like what?" (gesturing to draw/write on paper)

Step #3: Synthesizing

"And what do you know…now?" (gesturing to drawing)
"And what difference…does knowing that…make?"

If you have the participants share in groups of two or three, you could instruct them to take turns presenting their drawings to each other. Give each person one to two minutes to describe his drawing and then have the listeners use the following CLQ to help the speaker discover still more information:

"And what else do you know…about that?" (gesturing to the whole drawing or a specific detail)

(If you do this sharing, see the paragraphs on "After the guided process" at the beginning of this section again for instructions to listeners on "Facilitating tips.")

Examples

Three members of this workshop group have three entirely different goals, yet the facilitator poses the same questions to them all at the same time. Note: because this is just to give you a general idea of how this process could work, I am showing only one round of questions. Ideally, the facilitator would do six rounds before moving to Step #3: Synthesizing.

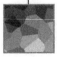

Remember: while the participants' answers are written out here, in a group session, participants would consider them silently, making notes or adding to their drawings as they wish.

Participant #1

Establishing what the client wants and a drawing: a Before Our Session sheet

#1:   *I want to have control of my anger.*

Drawing: large male lion tamer looks at a lion in cage

Initial round

Facilitator: **And as you look at what that would look like…,what are you drawn to?**

#1:   *I notice I'm on the outside of the cage and the lion is inside.*

Facilitator: **And what do you know…about that?**

#1:   *There is a door to the cage and it has a lock.*

Facilitator: **And that would look like what?**

#1 adds a padlock to the door latch.

Facilitator: **And what else do you know…about that?**

#1:   *I know that I hold the key to the cage. I can open it when I want the fuel anger gives me, and I can shut it when it threatens to overwhelm me.*

Facilitator: **And that would look like what?**

#1 adds a key hanging from lion tamer's belt.

(Imagine five repeated rounds.)

Synthesizing

Facilitator: **And when all that** (gesturing to drawing),**…what do you know…now?**

#1:   *I know that I am not my anger! I can control it; it is not who or what I am.*

Facilitator: **And what difference…does knowing that…make?**

#1:   *It means my anger may roar and try to sound big and dangerous, but I don't have to cower from it and let it take over.*

Facilitator: **And that would look like what?**

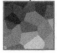

#1 adds colors to make the top hat deep black. He adds tails to the jacket and makes it bright red.

Participant #2

Establishing what the client wants and a drawing: a Before Our Session sheet

#2:   *I want to accept that I am single now and embrace living again.*

Drawing: a stick figure holds a bouquet of flowers

Initial round

Facilitator: **And as you look at what that would look like…,what are you drawn to?**

#2:   *I notice there are many different kinds of flowers. They have many colors: red, lavender, fuchsia, yellow.*

Facilitator: **And what do you know…about that?**

#2:   *They fill my arms. And my arms embrace them.*

Facilitator: **And that would look like what?**

#2 adds more flowers and traces over her arms and hands.

Facilitator: **And what else do you know…about that?**

#2:   *I know that just like I have to pay attention to really appreciate the flowers, to notice their colors and their smells and their variety, so I have to pay attention to what's around me, look for opportunities to find and get involved in wonderful things again.*

Facilitator: **And that would look like what?**

#2 adds flowers growing out of grass, off to figure's left and right. Takes care to have flowers be different colors and types.

(Imagine five repeated rounds.)

Synthesizing

Facilitator: **And when all that** (gesturing to drawing),**…what do you know…now?**

#2:   *I know now, not just rationally, but in a deeper sort of way, that I can't sit and wait for them to come to me. I have to go out and seek them and pick them. I have to act!*

Facilitator: **And what difference…does knowing that…make?**

#2:   *It sort of energizes me. Gardens energize me; so do flowers. They wake me up, engage me, and so can new things in my life if I just get outside of my little burrow!*

Participant #3

Establishing what the client wants and a drawing: a Before Our Session sheet

#3:   *I'd like to be the kind of parent my teenager can open up to.*

Drawing: Two stick figures sitting side by side in a car.

Initial round

Facilitator: **And as you look at what that would look like…,what are you drawn to?**

#3:   *That's my daughter in the passenger seat, and that's me, driving. My eyes are on the road ahead.*

Facilitator: **And what do you know…about that?**

#3:   *I notice I have big ears!* (laughs) *I guess I'm not looking at her, but I'm listening.*

Facilitator: **And what would look like what?**

#3 traces ears with dark lines.

Facilitator: **And what else do you know…about that?**

#3:   *I know that my daughter speaks up more when I'm not looking at her. I guess she feels less scrutinized.*

Facilitator: **And that would that look like what?**

#3 puts a cartoon bubble above daughter's head. Inside it says, "Dad, I was wondering about…"

(Imagine five repeated rounds.)

Synthesizing

Facilitator: **And when all that** (gesturing to drawing)**,…what do you know…now?**

#3: *I know I need to talk less and listen more, give her time and space to talk un interrupted. I know that for the future ahead…it's the time I give to really listen that will shape our relationship more than the advice.*

Facilitator: **And what difference…does knowing that…make?**

#3: *It means I can be more patient; I can keep my eye on the road ahead. I feel like my perspective has shifted. I'm thinking more long term: how this moment will serve the relationship I want to have with her in the long term… and not so much about what needs to happen in the next hour or day.*

The questions may not always correspond entirely logically with the information that individual participants may be thinking. No need to worry about it. People don't seem to mind; they adjust.

Working with a shared theme or issue

Individuals

Though you have a group of individuals working on their own self-development, your group may be organized around a particular issue: grief and loss, smoking cessation, addiction recovery, leadership development, anger management, self-esteem building, etc. If you decide to set some structure at the outset to keep everyone working on a particular theme, you can adapt your instructions on the Before Our Session sheet with more specific wording:

> **"What would you like to have happen *in regard to [x]*?"**

Examples

> **What would you like to have happen in regard to** your family?
>
> **What would you like to have happen in regard to** your illness?
>
> **What would you like to have happen in regard to** finding your purpose?
>
> **What would you like to have happen in regard to** working as a team?

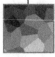

Aim to use wording that is as brief and broad as possible, allowing each person to individualize the issue he addresses. That way, you are meeting each person where he is at that moment. You could put your theme on a board or flip chart and have participants call out their answers to what they would like to have happen in regard to it while you or a scribe writes them down for all to see. This way, you can be sure your group members have the idea of stating a *want* (as opposed to focusing on a problem, for example), and they might get some ideas from each other. Once you have collected a good number of suggestions, encourage each person to silently select the words he wants to use—from the list or not—and fill in his Before Our Session sheet.

This way, you can simply gesture toward the list when you come to saying "that" in the script.

Another option is to adapt this question, developed by Clean therapists Caitlin Walker and Dee Berridge, on your Before Our Session sheet:

> **"When you're [x-ing] at your best,…that's like what?"**

Examples

> **When you're** counseling/coaching **at your best,…that's like what?**
>
> **When you're** learning **at your best,…that's like what?**
>
> **When you're** concentrating **at your best,…that's like what?**
>
> **When you're** connecting **at your best,…that's like what?**

Collaborative group

You can use this same approach for a collaborating team when your goal is to have the members learn more about themselves as individuals and about each other. Having greater insight into each other's fundamental perspectives and priorities can result in better team work, whatever the context.

Group therapy

The processes described in this book are meant for panning for gold. While therapists may well feel the need to be more directive than these processes, I suggest you give them a try without "adding to." In a group therapy context, they may be useful as a way to help group members get to know one another in the early stages or as a prompt to gather material to be worked with further. We say in the poetry therapy community, "Metaphors conceal and reveal and heal." Talking about what something *is like* for you rather than what it actually *is* provides some privacy and a feeling of safety while still addressing core issues. Group members can easily find their individual metaphors when they draw. And people tend to really like talking about them!

FAQs | *Frequently Asked Questions*

What's a good way to have all members share their results with a large group?

I can appreciate that for the sake of a sense of community or therapeutic intentions, it may not be satisfactory to have sharing only in small groups. If you have too large a group or too short a time period for everyone to hear each other out, consider having all members put their metaphor maps up on the walls or in the center of the floor, and give the group members time to walk around and look them over. Particularly if your group is organized around a particular theme, be it conflict resolution or confidence building, for example, seeing other maps even without hearing explanations of them, is likely to be a powerful experience for all.

The group members as a whole can be invited to share their comments on the *process* of exploring their metaphors. You could pose the question "*Without discussing content, what was this experience like for you?*" This is helpful for a group who may not want to share personal information. It also provides a way for everyone to feel heard without taking up the time to hear everyone's story.

Still, be prepared as a facilitator for some people to start telling their stories at length, monopolizing the group's time. Determine in advance how you will handle this. Indulging one person can lead to an avalanche of detail from those who come next!

Speaking of personal information…

Sometimes deeply personal and emotional things come up for participants. In a workshop group, for example, it may not be appropriate for an individual to share this kind of information. You have to help with this situation, for it may seem like a good idea to the participant in the heat of the moment, but later he may regret having shared such personal information with people he may not know well and actually become more guarded rather than more open. Then again, if it is a group of people he will likely never see again, they could be just the people he wants to share with.

It's tricky, and I suggest you give thought ahead of time to what seems right for your context and contract with your participants. What have they signed up for? A creative writing experience? Then try not to let it get into intensely therapeutic territory. A personal journey retreat? Then likely they have different expectations. Is it a group in school? Since it is best to assume confidentiality will *not* be maintained, I would keep a tight rein on what is shared. Consider your group's purpose and your training. While I do not like to encourage you to substitute your judgment for your adult clients—that does not seem very Clean—and I do not mean to suggest you should run fearfully from every revelation—you are the one setting up the conditions for growth and healing. You

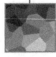

need to think about keeping your group members "safe," both in the moment and later. Perhaps you will want to set some parameters for the group about what is appropriate for sharing before you start inviting participants to speak. Even with that, have some statement you can calmly deliver should someone start to stray. Decide whether you will state it as a question, offering a choice (as in this example), or as a statement. And be sure to include an alternative or redirect so the person doesn't simply feel silenced.

Just one possible wording:

"This is starting to sound deeply personal, (name). Is this something you want to share here, or might this better be shared in private? Perhaps you could talk about what the experience of finding your metaphors was like for you?"

Then again, if you are running a group therapy program, you may be delighted to hear that this kind of in-depth sharing can be fostered with this Clean group process.

What I am going to describe in detail now is another lean Clean process, our 12th and last in the book. It is designed for a group whose members collaborate with one another. Whether you are facilitating two people or as many as sixteen, you can use this Clean process. I first learned it in 2003 from James Lawley and Penny Tompkins, who worked with Caitlin Walker on refining her design of this process, based on what became part of her Metaphors at Work methodology (Walker, 2014).

PROCESS #12: CLEAN GROUP METAPHOR MAP

Designed to:

Help group members know one another better
Help group members find common ground and purpose
Develop a common language to talk about an issue with
Better understand group members' different perspectives, priorities, working styles, etc.
Improve group function

Useful for:

Groups with 2–16 participants:
Couples/families
Workshops for groups
Businesses/team management
Organizational boards
Planning committees
Student groups
Teams

Time to allot: Varies depending on the size of the group; a couple might need only 10 minutes; a large group might need an hour.

Materials needed: Plain paper and markers

Clean Group Metaphor process

Setup

- Before a group starts working with this process, you will want to lay the groundwork.

- Talk about what it means to listen, question, and share Cleanly.

- Write "And is there anything else about that [x]?" on the board or flip chart where everyone can see it. Teach everyone how to ask this CLQ so that group members can further develop their understanding of their own and each other's ideas.

- Provide a simple stick-figure drawing and demonstrate asking the above CLQ and answering it. Modeling this for a large group will help give individuals an idea of an appropriate length answer. Your simple drawing will also ease some people's anxieties about coming up with a "good drawing."

- Let group members know they will need a timekeeper and a spokesperson for the group at various points along the way and that they need not be the same people the whole time.

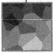

Step #1: Determine what the group wants

Depending on the context, the topic may be supplied by:

- you
- the group leader or manager (if it is someone other than you)
- group consensus

The group needs a clear, concise sentence [x] that answers this question:

> **"And what would you like to have happen?"**

Examples of group goals:

- Determine our most effective management style
- Have a smoothly functioning, happy classroom
- Have our family members treat each other with respect
- Work better as a team
- Allow each other to grieve as he needs to

Step #2: Get individual metaphor maps of the goal

Invite participants to *draw* their version of the goal by asking:

> **"And [x] would look like what?"**

Step #3: Present metaphor maps in small groups

Depending on the size of the group and the time you have, you may need to divide participants into smaller groups to share. A general guideline: try to have no more than four to a group. Have each participant present his drawing with a brief explanation.

If you are working in multiple, smaller groups, be sure each group elects a timekeeper. Give clear directions as to how much time each person has to describe his drawing (say, perhaps, one to two minutes), and have each timekeeper determine a gentle signal for "time's almost up." People get very involved in talking about something so personal to them, and they can really eat up your allotted time.

After the person's time is up, other participants can ask a few Clean questions to get still more information. One question per group member **"And is there anything else about [y = questioner's choice of exact word/phrase]?"** will probably be all you have time for if each group has three or more participants.

If group members ask you for more detailed instructions, just shrug vaguely and let them know they can work things out for themselves as long as they (1) stay Clean and (2) include everyone.

Step #4: Merging metaphor maps

Group members create a new metaphor map representing the group's metaphor for the goal. *At least one element* needs to be included from each participant's drawing. And everyone should be satisfied that his important wants and needs are represented in the new map.

You may want to post this question somewhere where the group can refer to it if there is a dilemma:

> **"What needs to happen in your group's drawing for your want/need/understanding to be represented?"**

Once the group has created its new metaphor map, the members should select a spokesperson to represent their group in the next step.

Step #5: Merging group metaphor maps

Now two groups will join together. A spokesperson for each group presents his group's metaphor map (note: each member *does not* review his original drawing, as it is included in the group's joint drawing). The combined group will now go through the same process, creating a single metaphor map that represents key concepts of both metaphor maps. There should be at least one element from each group's map in the new one.

The groups will continue this process until everyone is working together in one group to create a final group metaphor map.

Step #6: Synthesizing

You are giving the group members a chance to consider what they know now and the difference that makes. Decide, given your time and intent, how participants will share their answers to these questions and where to go from there. Will you give quiet time for writing? Will you share these results as a group, perhaps asking Clean questions of the comments? Will you do a go-round with everyone having a turn to speak? How will you record the answers? Who will use the notes and to do what? Will you do a Clean Action plan? It will all depend on your context, what you want to accomplish, and input from the group members.

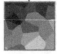

Trouble shooting

Having trouble getting the group to agree on a goal? You might want to consider having the group work with this [x]:

"We'd like to be able to agree on a common goal."

In going through the process, aspects of working together will reveal themselves, which may prove to be an excellent way to identify what a useful common goal they could work on might be.

Option: Combine Steps #1 and #2

Another way to address the issue is to provide the group with a goal determined by you or by the person in charge of the group in, for example, a professional context. While it would be ideal—and certainly Cleaner—to allow the group members to determine what their goal needs to be, sometimes time or purpose just does not allow for it.

Since the question provides the goal, this asks for a drawing:

"And when we're [x-ing] at our best, that would look like what?"

Examples of [x-ing]

1. Communicating
2. Parenting
3. Supporting each other
4. Exploring new ideas
5. Finding a common goal to agree on

Clean Group Metaphor Map script

Step #1: Establishing the goal

Group is provided with or selects a single goal [x] that answers the question,

> **"And what would you like to have happen?"**

Step #2: Creating a metaphor map

Each individual does a drawing representing his answer to the question,

> **"And [x] would look like what?"**

Step #3: Present to group

Each participant presents his metaphor map. Other participants ask a few Clean questions of some exact words ([y]) the drawing creator used, or they can simply gesture to something on the page. CLQ:

> **"And is there anything else about that [y]?"**

Step #4: Merging metaphor maps

Each small group creates a single drawing that includes at least one element from every participant's drawing. Remind participants of this next question if it is needed:

> **"And what needs to happen in your group's drawing for your want/need/understanding to be represented?"**

Step #5: Merging group metaphor maps

Repeat Steps #3 and #4, having the larger groups now present to each other, merge their ideas into a new drawing, and present to the next group pairing.

Step #6: Synthesizing

The groups keep repeating Step #5 until the whole group has a single metaphor map. The facilitator reviews key words the participants used to describe this final metaphor map and then asks:

> **"And what do you know…now?"**
>
> **"And what do you know now…about [x]?"**
>
> **"And what difference…does knowing that…make?"**

Thus, the whole process would look like this:

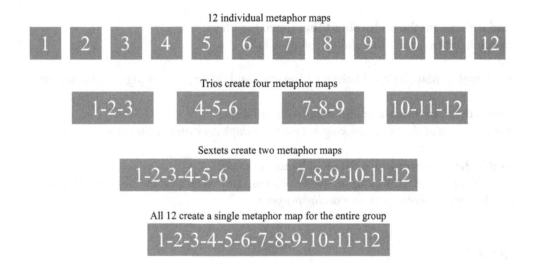

12 individual metaphor maps

| 1 | 2 | 3 | 4 | 5 | 6 | 7 | 8 | 9 | 10 | 11 | 12 |

Trios create four metaphor maps

| 1-2-3 | 4-5-6 | 7-8-9 | 10-11-12 |

Sextets create two metaphor maps

| 1-2-3-4-5-6 | 7-8-9-10-11-12 |

All 12 create a single metaphor map for the entire group

1-2-3-4-5-6-7-8-9-10-11-12

Example: Team work

The CEO of a small company expresses frustration with two departments in her company. Relationships between team members are testy, and they are not sharing and communicating as the boss wants them to. Her goals: increase the mutual respect and understanding that members of the two departments have for one another and improve their willingness to share information and function together for the good of the company.

Step #1: Determining the goal

The facilitator and CEO work out this goal statement incorporated into a directive:

> Working together at our best as one team **would look like what?**

Step #2: Individual metaphor maps

Four members from Department A are paired up with four members of Department B. First, each employee comes up with his own metaphor map in answer to the question posed. Then he describes it to his partner. The other member of the pair twice selects words/phrases the describer used and asks, **"And is there anything else about that [y]?"**

Pair A

#1 Metaphor Map: A mountain-climbing team is making its way up a tall mountain. The team members' task is to reach the top. That's their goal, and their greatest challenge.

And is there anything else about that climbing?
The climbers are roped together, helping pull each other up.

And is there anything else about that roped together?
They also protect each other should someone fall.

#2 Metaphor Map: It's an old-time sailing ship, and the crew is sailing it. All hands on deck!

And is there anything else about all hands on deck?
The captain is at the wheel, looking out over the ship's deck and at the ocean.

And is there anything else about all hands on deck?
Yes. There's a lookout way up in the crow's nest and other sailors manning the sails' ropes, which is vital to keeping them working properly.

Pair B

#3 Metaphor Map: It's a symphony orchestra. All the musicians are in their seats, playing music.

And is there anything else about that orchestra?
There are all these different sections: strings, winds, percussion, and so on. They're all needed if we're going to make beautiful music.

And is there anything else about they're all needed?
There's a conductor, and she's important, but so is the first violinist...so is each individual musician, because if anyone screws up, if anyone plays too loudly on his part or misses his entrance, then it's all messed up.

#4 Metaphor Map: It's a soccer team, all the players, offensive, defensive, the goalie. They're all there.

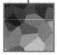

And is there anything else about all the players?
They're all different ages and have different degrees of experience, and that counts too. It's not just the youngest and fastest or the ones with the most endurance. Some contribute leadership and experience too.

And is there anything else about that experience?
They've got each other's backs. They know each other so well, it's almost intuitive. They compensate for each other's weaknesses; they know each other's strengths.

Pair C

#5 Metaphor Map: It's like a surgical team. Everyone has his role: the doctors, the nurses, the anesthesiologist. They're all needed to have the patient survive and get better.

And is there anything else about that surgical team?
There are people behind the scenes you don't see, but they're important too. If someone hadn't sterilized the room properly, the patient could get a deadly infection. Someone needs to keep the monitors running and accurate. There's a lot more to the operating room than you might think.

And is there anything else about that operating room?
There's music playing. It helps keep everyone calm and focused. It's about having the right atmosphere for the surgery too.

#6: Metaphor Map: It's like a bee colony. You have worker bees, drones, and the queen bee. This is their hive, with lots of little cells or compartments.

And is there anything else about that colony?
Bees have really sophisticated, complex social systems, with roles determined for each type of bee. And they have to function as a coordinated system.

And is there anything else about that coordinated system?
Bees depend upon chemical pheromones for communication and on a "dance" they do. Without being able to communicate, like where food sources are, they can't survive.

Pair D

#7 Metaphor Map: It's like an old-fashioned clock mechanism, with lots of gears.

And is there anything else about those gears?
The gears are all different sizes, but they fit together, mesh perfectly.

And is there anything else about that mechanism?
There are other parts too. Screws and springs and little levers, parts I don't really know what they are or what they do, but they need to be there to make the clock work. 'Cause it can't just run; it has to keep accurate time to be of any use.

#8 Metaphor Map: It's a solar system. And there's its sun in the middle.

And is there anything else about that system?
There are planets, lots of sizes, and some have their own moons orbiting them. And some have rings around them.

And is there anything else about those planets?
They're all orbiting the sun. That's their function, their part in the system. Get far enough away, and you can't even tell how one orbit relates to the other, but they all have their particular speed, direction, spinning, and so on. There's a master plan that keeps it all functioning as a system.

Could you have imagined so many different metaphors for working together as a team? Now the pairs' job is to combine their two very different metaphors into one picture. Personalities and group dynamics inevitably affect the outcome. The CEO watches, making mental notes about how her employees work with one another. The process itself is revealing, and everyone is likely to learn something from it.

Don't be surprised if some of the combined maps leave out what *you* might think was key information or have funny elements or plays on words emerge. (Part of what makes this a team-building exercise is that people generally have fun doing it!) Some maps may be dominated by one person's vision with only hints of the second person's input. Some might have new elements or images that were in neither original metaphor map. It is all part of the process.

Step #2: Presenting to the other groups

This is how the group spokespeople described their combined metaphor maps.

#1 and #2 had the mountain-climbing team and the sailing ship crew.

Their metaphor map shows six people on the sailing ship, making their way to the mountain. Two team members are already on the mountain and have set up a base camp. Once the team members arrive on the ship, the captain and the head of the mountaineers will study their maps and determine the best route to scale the mountain. All eight members on the mission will take the ropes from the sails and use them as climbing ropes.

#3 and #4 had the symphony orchestra and the soccer team.

Their new map shows an orchestra whose members are all wearing soccer uniforms with their numbers and names prominently on display. Some players have their eyes closed, listening intently and staying with the others, using their intuition. #3 really liked the idea of incorporating intuition as an important part of their vision, and everyone liked that. The conductor is conducting, and his musical score has both music on it and the score of the soccer game.

#5 and #6 had the surgical team and the bee colony.

Five bees stand around an operating table, dressed in surgical masks and gowns. On the table is the queen bee, wearing a crown. They are taking care of her, keeping track of her vitals on a monitor behind them. Three bees stand off to the side, vibrating their wings very fast. This is keeping the room comfortably cool and is also creating a pleasant hum, like music.

#7 and #8 had the clock mechanism and the solar system.

The new map is of a solar system. #7 liked the idea of the planets that have some more space between them, that aren't as closely enmeshed as clock gears. He felt the solar system also has his concept of accurate timing being important. So what is #7's contribution to the metaphor map? Saying they had to follow the rules to have something of #7's included, the pair added some "mysterious" screws and springs orbiting the planets, whose purpose neither #7 nor #8 know, describing themselves as pleased with the mystery of these parts.

I trust by now that you get the idea. For the next round, #1–#4 get together, present their two maps to each other, and make a single metaphor map. #5–#8 do the same. Those two groups then present their two maps and combine them to create one single group metaphor. So what might the final merged map look like?

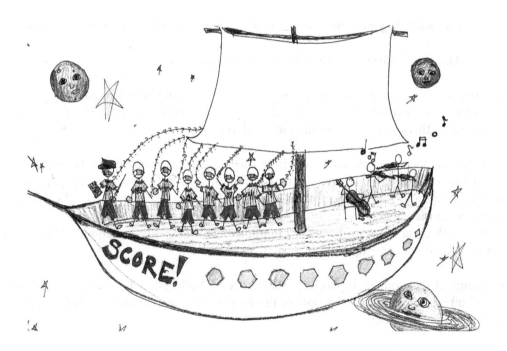

The group's metaphor

The final metaphor map depicts a spaceship with sails. There are rows of portholes along the side that look like honeycomb cells. The eight crew members are on deck, wearing soccer uniforms and surgical masks. Each one has a cell phone, also shaped like a honeycomb cell, so they can communicate with every other crew member. They hold ropes made of small linked question marks (to represent the mysterious unknown, they say) attached to the sails. The captain wears a hat with gold braid on it and carries a map and baton. The ship, whose name "Score" is painted along its hull, sails among the planets, each of which has eyes and a nose and mouth, suggesting human qualities. On deck is a string quartet, playing the score of *2001: A Space Odyssey.*

As you can tell, a metaphor landscape does not necessarily follow the rules of physics or logic. It will not matter to the group one bit. I think of the metaphors as having their own *dream logic.*

Final assessments

With a group metaphor map now on display, individual participants are asked to return to their original places and take some time to write their answers to these last three questions, which are posted where everyone can see them. They are told that they will each be called upon to share *something* with the group, but they will not be required to share everything they write.

"And what do you know...now?"

"And what do you know now...about working together at our best as one team**?"**

"And what difference...does knowing that...make?"

Once response time is up, each person is given about a minute to pick something to share from what he has written. Everyone is told up front that no comment is to be made about what is said in this go-round other than to thank the person for sharing.

The group members are next asked to decide what actions they will take to "work together at their best as a team," and a lively discussion follows. They brainstorm a lengthy list of possible actions and vote on their top four choices. The eight participants are divided into four teams consisting of a member from each department and tasked to return the following week with suggestions for next steps to implement their assigned actions. (They could use Clean Action to come up with these steps.)

The picture of the group metaphor is posted above the coffeepot, where it can be seen and enjoyed often, reminding participants of the good time they had and the new metaphor vocabulary they now share.

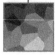

FAQs | *Frequently Asked Questions*

This process sounds like it could take a fair amount of time. What am I supposed to be doing?

Your job as facilitator of the process is to hold the space and to keep people on task and asking Clean questions of each other, which encourages listening respectfully and accurately.

What if group members start arguing?

Should tempers flare as some group members try to negotiate what gets on to the group map, try to stay out of it. If the group calls you over, you could listen to the spokesperson and ask of each person in the group,

> **"And what would you like to have happen?"**

If you feel you must intervene more to keep the group as a whole moving along, pose a different Clean question and model calm curiosity. Besides suggestions made in the script, you could ask,

> **"And is there anything in your drawing that is *like* this other drawing?"**

Notice this question is directed toward the *drawings*, not the individuals who made them. Keeping the attention off the people and on the metaphors creates some separation between the concepts and the people who came up with them. This is one of the values of the process.

The goal is to foster *group ownership* of the metaphor map. Once the groups get to the first round of combined metaphors, everyone has given up something and had something of his included, so feathers that have been ruffled usually start to smooth out.

And if they don't? The process of condensing metaphor maps to a single group map can be very revealing as to the patterns certain group members bring to the group dynamic. In a therapeutic context, this can suggest where attention might next be focused, whether it is having the group identify what works well or what does not. For business or educational groups with deadlines and goals to be met and with some flexibility as to who is assigned to work with whom, it may become clearer what team changes need to be made. The saboteur, the leader, the compromiser, the rescuer, the nurturer, the bully, and so on all start to show their strengths and weaknesses.

Outcomes of developing a group metaphor

What happens *as* the group metaphor is created is sometimes the most helpful outcome.

Participants have heard…and seen…
> how other group members think
> what they value
> how they prioritize
> the group dynamic in an atypical context (potentially revealing unknown strengths, tensions, problems, possibilities)

Participants have
> felt heard
> felt included
> enjoyed each other

Participants have been encouraged to
> appreciate other's perspectives
> think imaginatively

This clarity and understanding can
> improve group dynamics
> enhance a sense of connection/community
> reveal what needs to change

Discussing a metaphor, rather than individuals, helps people feel
> safer
> less defensive
> more open to change

The group has a new shorthand

Taking advantage of the way a metaphor concisely packages a lot of information into a word or symbol, participants can now refer to any of the ones included in their group metaphor and convey a great deal of information. For example, a team leader who says, "*I need you manning the engine room while I'm at the helm*," may convey a great deal to the listener in a way that honors his participation in and understanding of the group's own language. The same can be true for a couple or family. Or a classroom group. Or any group whose functioning together can be made better with mutual understanding and respect.

Possibilities for using a group metaphor

These possibilities are limited only by your imagination! What has been described above is primarily for developing clarity and fostering community. You can certainly combine this process with others to fit your group's needs.[10]

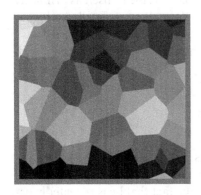

Mix and Match

CHOOSING A CLEAN PROCESS

So now you have 12 Clean processes to choose from. How do you decide which one to use with a client? There is no one right answer. Consider your client's strengths, weaknesses, preferences, your own intuition, and the time available.

Draw on strengths

One approach is to select a process that plays to your client's strength or preference, one you may observe or that the client tells you about. Your client may describe himself as artistic. Use metaphor maps. Or he may say he loves to dance or describe himself as primarily kinesthetic. Pick a spatial process such as Clean Networks. Your client may tell you he has ADHD (Attention Deficit Hyperactivity Disorder). He may well do better moving about so he does not have to sit in one place for very long. Think of his kinesthetic engagement with the world as a strength, and use it!

Enhance areas of weakness

You could take the opposite approach and choose a process that draws on an aspect of a client that he is less apt to choose. Find out what happens when he approaches his issues from a different modality. Part of his stuck-ness may come from the fact that he is repeatedly using the same internal process or perspective to address issues.

For a very verbal client or one who describes himself as usually being "in his head," any of the processes we have covered in this book will provide you with a helpful alternative to talk-only approaches.

What I am *not* suggesting is that you push a client to "overcome" or try to "get around" what you might be tempted to label as resistance. If your client does not want to address something or try a new process, honor that. In some deep way, his system knows he is not ready to go there or do that.

I do find some clients baulk at the idea of doing a drawing. They may say they are not artistic and get flustered. Use a light touch, add some humor, stress that stick-figure drawing is fine, that this is not about "making Art with a capital A." And if your client still doesn't want to draw, try something else. He may change his mind later.

Since all the Clean processes are just various ways of getting at some inner information, you needn't get too attached to using any one process over another. Go with the flow.

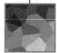

Think metaphorically

A person who describes himself as *stuck in place*, unable to take another perspective or make any sort of move to change, might benefit from getting up out of his seat and *moving*. Try Clean Space or Clean Networks. Or throw in a Clean Spinning set of questions; it will take only a few minutes, and you might just find your client loosens up to new possibilities or shifts direction. A client who says he is "painting himself into a corner" may benefit from a drawing process…or from a spatial process that includes a corner of the room. Listen to your client's metaphors!

Variety is the spice of life

Another way to decide what process to employ would be to do something different from what you have done before. If you have used movement techniques before, try drawing or vice versa. Your client may access different information or experience it differently. And many clients like to try new and/or different approaches. It keeps them curious, engaged, and committed. And it just might energize you too!

Abandoning a process

Sometimes you pick a process, and the client just doesn't get information from that way of working. I do not think it has ever happened with a client of mine before, but wouldn't you know, it happened just the other day. Steve had been talking about leaving a job that had been stressful for some time. I decided to try Clean Spinning to see whether turning in a different direction, presumably considering different perspectives, would be helpful.

What he got from the first two directions was vague and seemingly useless. He did face one direction from where he could "see a way out, a way forward," which sounded promising to me. But a follow-up question or two brought no more information, and he started to seem frustrated, said he was lost, couldn't find more answers, and lost his mindful focus, looking directly at me.

Now this is a moment of decision for a facilitator. Do I stay with what is happening in the moment, with "lost" or use CLQs to develop this client's phrase "a way out"? I took into account that (1) I was intending to pan for gold, not dig deeply in any one area, at least not at the start, and (2) Steve's body language was signaling he was disengaging from the process. I decided to abandon the Clean Spinning set of questions. Since a spatial technique did not seem helpful in that moment, I segued into a Clean Hiero session. Starting with written words seemed a more comfortable "way in" for Steve, and he went on to have a productive session.

Was that the right thing to do? Did I bail just at the point where frustration was ready to give way to new learning? Who knows? There probably wasn't one "right thing to do." I figure if my client is engaged with whatever process we are doing and getting information, then I have probably made a right choice. If after repeated tries, he is not, then I move on.

What if your client's inability to get information flowing is not about the process but what you might call his resistance?

One of the advantages of these panning for gold Clean processes is that clients quickly get the idea that (1) you are not going to be asking lots of questions about any one thing and (2) they are in control of what gets talked about and how much gets said, so the processes are not likely to trigger a lot of defensiveness. That is why I am more likely to think it is the process that is not working for the client.

But if your client reacts with what some professionals would label resistance, so what? Consider resistance to mean that the client is not ready to go where you are trying to guide his attention to go, so honor that and meet him where he is; do something else. What is he drawn to now?

Mix and match

Once you become comfortable and adept with these 12 lean Clean processes, you will find that they work together very well, which is hardly surprising since they all use Clean questions that have similar syntax, vocabulary, and rhythms and have evolved from Grove's same basic theory of how to help people self-explore.

I think of the mix and match processes you can use as falling into three categories:

- **Sequencing:** one process follows another in a session
- **Blending:** Clean questions from various processes are interwoven in small chunks throughout a session
- **Integrating:** Clean questions or processes are partnered with another methodology

SEQUENCING CLEAN PROCESSES

As I have mentioned in a number of places, when introducing these 12 processes, some of them naturally segue into one another in a logical sequence. For example, you select a way to prime the pump, follow it with one of the space or drawing processes, and end with one of the closure methods. This book is organized in sections to help you plan just this sort of sequencing. With the clients I have used multiple times for examples—such as Jaime—I have already demonstrated to you how you can sequence processes.

Having a plan

Sometimes you can make a pretty generic plan, like the sequence of three Clean processes in this next example, and stick to it. This is especially true if you are a counselor who may see a client only once or twice and have specific goals you are expected to accomplish. For example, you might be a career counselor or a therapist in a college counseling office, and insurance or your institution's rules will allow only one or two visits. Or you are doing an initial assessment of a client and want to get a general overview. You might also stick to such a plan if you are introducing Clean Language to a client and want to familiarize him with such experiences and/or specific processes.

It is also the way you may work when you are first learning these processes. Give yourself a break and choose a logical sequence to stick to so you will not be distracted by worrying about which process to choose in the moment or being competent with all the processes. Might there be a better selection you could have used? Maybe. But your client will still get something useful out of the session. Be patient with yourself as you learn. Your client won't know you have other options.

Responding to the moment

At other times, rather than depending on a predetermined sequence of Clean processes, it is the information that your client presents that will suggest which Clean process to use. (You may want to make a copy of the appropriate scripts at the back of the book to follow along with these examples, imagining you are facilitating. It will reinforce your learning of the scripts.)

Example #1: Clean Language/Metaphor Maps…Clean Boundaries…Group Metaphor

Jesse and Chris are seeking counseling because their marriage is in trouble. As their facilitator, I decide to start with Clean Language questions to encourage the couple to explore their metaphors with one another. This will help them know themselves and each other better. (I will not include all the questions and answers here, just enough so you can follow the process and the clients' maps.)

I go over how they will be using drawings to explore the metaphors that describe their relationship and what they want out of it and how it will help them know themselves and each other better. I point out the paper and the markers and give my usual bit about stick-figure drawings being fine. I want to get these logistical items out of the way before the couple gets into their stuff.

Facilitator: **And what would you like to have happen?**

Both Jesse and Chris agree they want to improve their marriage. They talk for a bit about how their marriage would be if it were improved. We join the session as the couple is agreeing on their goal.

We want to be there for each other, work together as a team.

I now have them do what the bottom part of a Before Our Session sheet directs them to do—make drawings.

Facilitator: **And that would look like what?** (gesturing to paper and markers)

Once they finish sketching, I let Jesse and Chris know that I will invite them both to describe their drawings. I add some Clean Language questions to develop more details so the describers can learn more about themselves as they speak and the partners can hear more about each other's world.

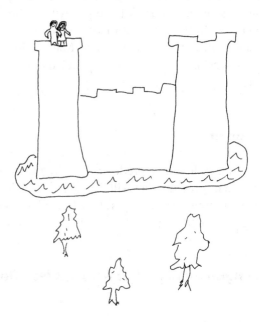

Facilitator: **And what's there?** (gesturing to drawing)

Jesse: *We're in a fortress surrounded by a moat, and she's at the top of a tower with me, on guard. And I know she's always got my back.*

Facilitator: **And is there anything else about that** fortress?

Jesse: *Yes, it's like those medieval ones, made of big, heavy stones with the round towers on the corners with those notches you can look between and still be safe...or at least, safer.*

It's Chris's turn now.

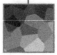

Facilitator: **And what's there?**

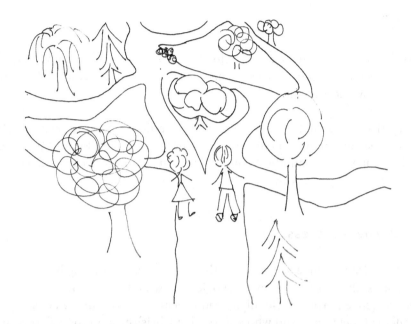

Chris: *We're walking together on a path in a beautiful grassy park with shade trees. And we walk together sometimes, and we go on separate paths sometimes, and then we come back to the same path again and walk for a while more together, holding hands. There are many paths going off in many directions.*

Facilitator: **And** many paths going off in many directions. **And what kind of** going off **is that** going off?

Chris: *It's an easy going off, a just-the-next-step sort of going off.*

I lay index cards on the table with the drawings that have on them the Clean Language questions I just used (What Kind of…, Anything else…) and have Chris and Jesse ask each other for more details. Not only am I helping them verbalize more information, but both partners learn something about listening without steering the conversation to himself or herself.

Chris: **And is there anything else about that** always got your back?

Jesse: *That's really the core of the whole thing: as a team, I need to know that's your top priority, that you've got my back, that the ring around us is secure.*

They switch roles.

Jesse: **And** go on separate paths sometimes. **And what kind of** separate **is that** separate?

Chris: *It's an easy-apart, easy-together kind of separate, like water flowing around a rock. It just goes around it and meets again on the other side. So we're walking together on the path again.*

Revealing questions

Notice that having the partners ask questions of each other reveals something about the partner asking the question too. Where is his or her attention and concern? What does she or he want to know more about?

You may find that you do not want to leave all the questions up to the partners. Maybe you will use a set of six questions structure: each partner asks six questions of the other's statements. If all is going well, go another round. Or *you* can ask more Clean Language questions or go on to another Clean process.

Segue to the next process

I decide to use Clean Boundaries, particularly because Jesse's drawing has such clearly defined boundaries (the fortress, the moat). Logically, I would expect the boundaries to serve important protective purposes. He might find it helpful to consider what is beyond them from the safety of metaphor. And who knows what Chris's exploration will reveal?

I am going to smoothly segue into Clean Boundaries without an announcement. My clients will not know one process has ended and another has begun; they do not need to. I start with Chris. I will let Jesse have a chance to see her go first and know what he can expect. I anticipate he might feel uneasy exploring beyond his protective boundaries, and I can at least reduce any qualms he may have about the process itself.

Chris has identified the initial space—a path. I pick up from there by asking about the boundary that defines the object.

Facilitator: (gesturing toward the path in her drawing) **And** walking together on the path. **And what kind of boundary does that** path **have?**

Chris: *That path has a distinct edge, like it used to be edged there down to the dirt and now the weeds have filled in the space.*

Facilitator: **And that would look like what?**

Chris adds some weeds and dots of dirt and darkens a line of the edge of the path and adds another line on the other side of the weeds.

Facilitator: **And what kind of space is beyond that?** (gesturing to *distinct edge*)

Chris: *That's where the grass starts. It's really pretty, very green grass.*

Facilitator: **And that would look like what?**

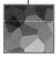

Chris takes her time adding grass with a green marker.

Facilitator: **And where does that space go?**

Chris: *As far as I can see, until it disappears over the hill…about a quarter of a mile away.*

Facilitator: **And what kind of boundary does that space have?**

Chris: *Oh, wow. Then there's a cliff!*

Chris reaches for another piece of paper and draws a cliff on the left side of the page. She puts the paper about a foot from her first drawing.

Facilitator: **And** a cliff! **And what kind of space is beyond that?** (gesturing to the *cliff*)

Chris: *Oh, it's an ocean. A vast and boundless ocean.*

Facilitator: **And** the vast and boundless ocean. **And that would look like what?**

I gesture toward her drawing, and she takes up markers again to add an ocean below the cliff.

Facilitator: **And where does that space go?**

Chris: *Almost as far as the human mind can conceive of.*

I want to take care here to slow down, to give Chris a chance to conceive of something so vast. So I hold her attention there with another CLQ.

Facilitator: **And is there anything else about** almost as far as the human mind can conceive of?

Chris: *It's an enormous expanse of ocean, as deep as it is wide.*

Facilitator: **And what kind of boundary does that space have?**

Chris: *It's where the Infinite begins its total blackness.*

Facilitator: **And** the Infinite…and total blackness. **And that would look like what?**

Chris looks around. Then she takes two more pieces of paper and blackens both with the marker. She puts her cliff and ocean drawing in the middle of four.

Facilitator: **And where does that space go?** (gesturing to the black pages)

Chris: *Beyond any papers I could put here. I can't see; it's like it's convex. It turns back again, like one of those infinity strips. Like that's its edge. Huh! Who knew?* (laughs)

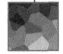

Think her science is a bit confusing here? Should you say something? Correct her? Absolutely not! These are her words, her vision. Stay Clean. You could ask a "What kind of?" or "Anything else?" question or let it ride. It is that dream logic that a metaphor landscape can have. Listen for *its* intrinsic logic, not the real world's.

Notice, I did not make the assumption that reaching a *boundless* ocean was the final frontier. Or the *Infinite*. Nor would I have stopped with a *turning back*. Maybe she would have gone on. Or maybe she would have said that was it. The point is, do not stop because your logic tells *you* it sounds like your client has reached an end point.

And do not expect spaces to always reach a cosmic scale like Chris's. There could be six types of spaces between here and the other side of a room! But at some point, you need to stop to keep the spaces a manageable number, keeping the whole of the session in mind.

By this time, Chris is getting the hang of this pattern of questions, and she describes the edge without being asked: it is convex. I choose not to ask for more details. I could go on to more spaces, but I have a second client to consider. One option is to complete Chris's Clean Boundaries process by leading her in reverse through her spaces, but Jesse has been waiting and watching for some time now. I leave Chris's system to percolate a bit with its new information and turn my attention to Jesse.

Switching partners

I start asking Jesse questions about his fortress metaphor. Some exploring about just how threatening the outside world is now could give his system some useful information. And it will probably be eye opening for Chris as well. I will repeat some of Jesse's words to get him back in touch with his drawing, encouraging him to psychoactive it again.

Facilitator:	(gesturing toward Jesse's drawing) **And** TEAM. **And** a fortress there. **And** a moat. **And what kind of a boundary does that** moat **have?**
Jesse:	*It's actually grassy right up to the edge of the moat.*
Facilitator:	**And where does that space go?**
Jesse:	*Oh, maybe 100 yards in all directions.*
Facilitator:	**And that would look like what?**

Jesses fills in the area around the moat with green marker some four to six inches out.

Facilitator:	**And what kind of boundary does that space have?**
Jesse:	*There are woods that start right here from the edge of the grass.*

Jesse has gotten the hang of it now. He doesn't wait for my prompt; he draws the woods.

Facilitator: **And what kind of space is beyond that boundary?** (gesturing to the trees along the edge of the grass)

Jesse adds some details to the edge of his woods with individual trees with different sorts of leaves. Then he starts making lots of dark, swirling shapes next to them that become indistinguishable from each another.

Jesse: *It gets dark very quickly once you enter the woods. Lots and lots of trees.*

Jesse's brow is furrowed, and he seems to be focused on this space with more intensity than he has shown so far. So I ask another CLQ.

Facilitator: **And is there anything else about that space?**

Jesse: *That's a disaster waiting to happen.*

Jesse adds more dark green color, his "tree tops" of green circles swirling into one another.

As I watch, it occurs to me that Jesse did not say a disaster *was* there but that it was waiting to happen. I ask one more CLQ to draw his attention to this and see what his system learns. Since we are panning for gold here, I will leave it to that one question and let Jesse just sit with his answer.

Facilitator: **And is there anything else about that** waiting to happen**?**

Jesse: *I guess disaster doesn't always come. Just sometimes.*

Facilitator: **And where does that space go?**

Jesse: *That's the unknown. You never know what might be in there, and you can't see to the end when you're in it. The trees are too thick.*

Facilitator: **And what kind of boundary does that space have?**

Jesse adds a wavy line about four inches into the woods.

Jesse: *It's wavy, like you can't quite tell where it is; it's mysterious, sort of. Like, where does the unknown actually stop?*

Facilitator: **And is there anything else about that** mysterious**?**

Jesse: *It's not under my control.*

Jesse takes his time, adding more swirls and wavy lines.

Facilitator:	**And what kind of space is beyond that?** (gesturing to the wavy lines)

Jesse: *They stop here. There's a clearing in the middle of the woods. A clearing with an old campfire circle in the middle, a ring of stones.*

Facilitator: **And that would look like what?**

Jesse: *The circle of stones is about two feet across, not all that big. Enough for a couple of people to gather around is all. A fire in there could keep a couple of people warm.*

The direction of the space's edges has stopped expanding and turned inward on itself. So I do a bit of repeating and ask a question to hold Jesse's attention here briefly. When we get back to him, I will reverse his direction to revisit his spaces.

Facilitator: **And what kind of** people **could those** people **be?**

Jesse: *Like Chris and me.*

Chris smiles, and Jesse returns her smile.

Switching back

As Jesse's attention has turned to Chris, it seems a particularly appropriate moment to move back to Chris's drawing. Time to revisit her spaces in reverse. Again, I repeat a few of her last words while gesturing to her drawing to get Chris back into her deeply mindful state of involvement with her metaphor landscape.

Facilitator: **And convex. And** turns back, like an infinity strip. **And what does that boundary know?** (gesturing to outermost boundary)

Chris: *Huh! Now it's like a mirror. A convex mirror. And everything reflected in it seems smaller, like it's not that big a deal. It knows, if you look at it from an other perspective, what Jesse and I are struggling with is not that big a deal, from the Infinite way of things.*

Now, I don't know what she means by the "Infinite way of things." I could ask another Clean Language question, thinking perhaps she could use some clarity too. But Chris seems satisfied with her answer, nodding her head. Since it is not about my understanding the point, I stay with the Clean Boundaries process. I will simply invite her to add to her drawing.

Facilitator: **And that would look like what?**

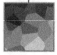

Chris adds a scrolled frame to her strip, like a mirror might have. I continue asking about the spaces and boundaries in reverse order, gesturing as I go to the appropriate image.

Facilitator: **And what does that space know?**

Chris: *The Infinite blackness is a place of rest. It knows we have to take time some times from working on our relationship to just be. To rest and just be.*

Facilitator: **And what does that boundary know?**

Chris: *It knows that journeys end and every life is a process of learning, of doing and being.*

Facilitator: **And what does that space know?**

Chris: *This is the ocean. It knows that things aren't always what they seem on the surface, that there's a lot of life in its depths.*

Because her answer suggests some new images, I invite Jaime to add details.

Facilitator: **And that would look like what?**

Chris adds what I take to be many fish and some coral.

Facilitator: **And what does that boundary know?**

Chris: *Ah, the cliff! The cliff knows that change can be intimidating. And it can also be exciting.*

Facilitator: **And what does that space know?**

Chris: *The grassy space knows that Jesse and I are a team, whether we sense it or not. We are always connected, and we have a lot of good history that binds us. It offers us many paths and many choices and much to share.*

Without a prompt, Chris traces over some of the path's lines and then looks up.

Facilitator: **And what does that boundary know?**

Chris: *This little space knows that we're just going through a little rough patch (tearing up). You know, when I first drew that, I was thinking that the weeds beside the path were about our relationship going to seed, sort of. But now I see that it wasn't that at all. This is such a small space compared to all the rest. I didn't realize that before.*

She reaches out for Jesse's hand, and he takes hers. I wait for their silent communication to end when Chris looks up again.

Facilitator:	**And what does the** path **know?**

Chris:	*That we're in this together, on this path together, no matter where we actually are* (as she gestures around her entire drawing).

Without prompting, she redraws the figures so that they are holding hands. I end this portion of the session with a Clean closure, a way to gently bring this mini session with Chris to a close.

Facilitator:	**And is there anything else about all...that for right now?**

Chris:	*No, it's good. In fact, it's* really *good.*

Taking turns

I return now to Jesse's drawing, repeating some of his words from the last space he discovered to get him in touch again with his metaphor landscape. Jesse did not end with a final edge but a circular fire, so I adjust my first question to suit the situation, skipping the first question about the outer boundary. Don't be a slave to the script! You have to follow the logic of what your client is saying.

I gesture to each space and boundary as I ask about it.

Facilitator:	**And** a fire that can keep a couple of people warm. **And what does that space know?**

Jesse:	*The fire knows that at the heart of it all, there is warmth and love.*

Facilitator:	**And what does that boundary know?**

Jesse:	*I put the stones there to keep the fire in, to contain it, to protect us both.*

Facilitator:	**And what does that space know?**

Jesse:	*It knows that sometimes there needs to be space and air for a fire to breathe.*

Facilitator:	**And what does that boundary know?**

Jesse:	*It knows for trees to thrive, there needs to be some clear space.*

Facilitator:	**And what does that space know?**

Jesse:	*It knows that though the woods can feel foreboding, there is life in the woods too. It's not just dark.*

Facilitator:	**And that would look like what?**

Jesse starts to add something to his dark green woods, but nothing can be seen. He looks around.

Jesse: *Do you have some scissors and tape?*

I always keep some at hand. Jesse draws birds and small animals and cuts them out. He tapes them onto the woods. When he's done, he smiles broadly.

Facilitator: **And what does that boundary know?** (gesturing to the edge of the woods)

Jesse: (smiles) *This boundary knows that transitions are not as extreme as they may look. Whether it's trees or grass, it's all plants; they're all growing.*

Facilitator: **And what does this space know?** (gesturing to the grass)

Jesse: *I'm not sure what it knows. It's like that's not important; it is just full of small, busy life, just being and growing and thriving. And getting sun, something about there being all the sun it needs.*

Facilitator: **And what does this boundary know?** (gesturing to the moat)

Jesse: *The moat knows it's about more than protecting our fortress. It's also about nurturing the life in it and in the grass. It holds life-giving water.*

Jesse adds what looks like geese or swans swimming in the moat.

Notice I asked about the boundary, and Jesse's answer was about the moat itself—a space. I do not go back; I follow his lead and his attention.

Facilitator: **And what does that boundary know?** (gesturing to the fortress wall)

Jesse: *That's the fortress wall. It knows it's strong. It knows it will stay strong and be there when it's needed, that I…that we don't have to be in it for it to be strong.*

Facilitator: **And what does that space know?** (gesturing to the whole fortress)

Jesse: *It's old…it's ageless. It has stood the test of time. It is confident it can withstand whatever.*

Facilitator: **And what do those words know?** (gesturing to TEAM)

Jesse: *They know…it's like they know they're alive again, revived like a plant that's been watered by the moat. There's a sort of organic quality to them now that's different. I can't really explain it.*

Facilitator: **And what do you know…now?**

Jesse: *I know that I am not as vulnerable as I thought I was, that fire and water and air and earth are all working together, just as they should.*

Facilitator: **And what do you know now about** "be there for each other" **and** "work together as a team"

Jesse: *I know that there are different ways and places to be there for each other and be a team. Either one of us could be the lookout, could raise or lower the water in the moat, could be sure the grass gets enough water. If it doesn't rain, we could put out sprinklers. We can both lay a fire or blow air on it to get it going. Whatever. Everything just feels like there's…I don't know…more air around everything now.*

Jesse now turns toward Chris, looking from her to her drawing. I return to Chris to ask the final questions of the Clean Boundaries process. (You do not have to split up the session questions this way; it is just one possibility. My reason for doing so was to avoid having Jesse wait too long without participating.)

Facilitator: **And** you're in this together, on this path together, no matter where you actually are. **And is there anything else that space knows?** (gesturing to the path where the two figures are)

Chris: *It knows the path can be easily widened or narrowed, and it's easy to add new paths. The paths knew all along; I thought it was harder than that.*

Facilitator: **And what do you know…now?**

Chris: *I just had no idea what Jesse was experiencing. I can't really say what his metaphors mean, but there was something about all that: the fortress, the moat, the fire…all of it. It was just really powerful.*

Facilitator: **And what difference…does knowing that…make?**

Chris: *I'm not sure yet. But it feels really important, like something shifted big time. And I realize I don't know Jesse as well as I thought I did. Which is kind of exciting, after all these years! Like there's still more to learn.*

Facilitator: **And what do you know now about** "be there for each other" **and** "work together as a team"**?**

Chris: *I have a lot more hope for us. And it doesn't seem like it will all be work. We can explore each other…like walking on a new path, but one I didn't anticipate at all, one we can walk together.*

Facilitator: **And is there anything else about all that…for right now?**

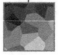

Jesse and Chris shake their heads and smile at each other.

Different styles

You may notice that Jesse stuck with talking about his metaphor landscape, whereas Chris spoke more literally in terms of their relationship. Expect that clients could do either or both. Just know that what you are hearing does not mean that Jesse is not also applying what he is noticing about his metaphors to his relationship nor that Chris's metaphors are not also evolving. Inevitably you, as a facilitator, are going to be privy to only some of what is going on.

Applying the group metaphor process to a couple

Chris and Jesse have about 15 minutes left at this point. As a way of bringing their two world visions together, I decide to use the Clean Group Metaphor Process. I invite the couple to take their individual images and create one drawing, a single vision of their original desire: to "be there for each other and work together as a team." The only guidelines I give are that their final drawing must include whatever aspects of the original metaphor landscape the creator feels is important to include, though it doesn't need to look like it does in the original drawing. And the final metaphor map must have at least one thing from each partner.

My intent is that once the couple discovers and shares a significant amount of information, they will likely better understand and appreciate the other's perspectives and needs. I anticipate they will be less likely to dismiss the symbols of the other ("Oh, we don't need a fortress. Nonsense.") after their experiences with Clean Language and Clean Boundaries. My intent is *not* to fix their relationship; whatever healing and growth occurs is up to Jesse and Chris.

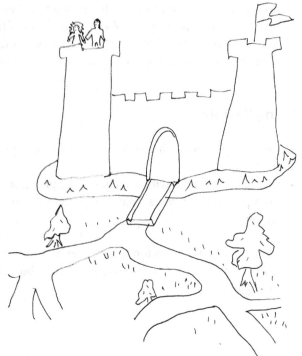

I leave them to it. I hear some questions from both about what the other wants to include. Both ask a "And what kind of..." CLQ once or twice, which gets them laughing.

What they come up with is a fortress with its drawbridge down, creating a path over the moat. On the other side is a grassy park with several paths. Both agree that they will have a flag to fly from the top of the tower that can be seen from all the paths. If a flag is flying, that means that one of them needs the other to come back to the fortress so they can pull up the drawbridge and help protect each other's back. Their new private catch phrase is "*The flag is flying.*"

Four simple words can now speak volumes. Time will tell whether knowing Jesse can communicate his needs easily and without drama or overtly admitting to what might feel to him like weakness means he can relax more about the times Chris is off on a separate path. Perhaps he will weather those times better knowing she is not abandoning her partner but just "*flowing around to the other side of a rock*," as she puts it. Or this is how I perceive it. But it is, after all, just my interpretation of what happened (rife with metaphors of my own, you may have noticed).

Things to consider

- Pay attention to the clock; you do not want to rush one process so that you can squeeze in another. One of your key roles as a facilitator of these processes is to hold the space and give your clients a chance to explore what is just on the tips of their conscious awareness. Feeling rushed will definitely interrupt the sort of mindful self-exploration you are trying to cultivate in your clients.

- There are all sorts of hard-to-quantify results these Clean processes may produce. Most likely, the sort of information clients will hear from their partners is not what they have ever shared before, and there will likely be surprises for both. Recognizing that their partner has an inner world of which they have been unaware returns some of the mystery of getting to know one another to the relationship. They are probably going to realize they made some assumptions about each other that are not true. Hmm…and is there anything else about *that*?

- My goal in the session above was not to have my clients leave with a single picture; it was to help them know and relate to one another better. It turned out they created one joint metaphor map as planned. Well and good. But if they had gotten no further than sharing their two separate maps, that would have been okay too. If they had baulked when asked to draw, I would have let go of my plan altogether and used another process.

Being flexible

In the example above, three Clean processes seamlessly flowed one into the next. Notice:

- Being Clean and having this book's 12 processes at the ready means that I do not stick to a plan for the plan's sake. I pay attention to what is happening in the moment and respond.

- You need to pay attention to any overlapping of CLQs when you sequence processes to avoid illogical repetition. No need to fret about it; this will seem natural when you are doing it!

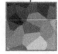

BLENDING CLEAN PROCESSES

Once you become really comfortable with these processes, you may find that you cherry-pick questions from them in response to what a client says or does rather than use an entire process. Nothing wrong with that as they are all Clean questions, but beware:

- These Clean processes are meant to pan for gold, not dig deeply. One of the reasons you have scripts is to keep the number of questions limited and to keep the client's attention moving rather than staying in any one place very long.

- Grove believed in the power of a set of six questions, the number he felt was the minimum to allow a deeper wisdom to emerge. If you do too much bouncing around (a Boundary question here, two Hiero questions there, a Networks question next), you may be pulling your client's attention in too many directions, too fast. It is about finding a fine balance: you don't want your questions to go too deeply, but neither should they be too scattered.

Given these considerations, what might a blended session sound like?

Let's start with a simple example. You can blend Clean Situating with some questions from Clean Start. The goal is to activate the client's intuitive knowing about what "feels right" and establish the optimal setup for your client to connect with his inner wisdom.

Example #2: Clean Situating…Clean Start

In this situation, you can think of the facilitator as the "object" whose position the client adjusts.

> **And where would you like to be?**
>
> **And where would you like me to be?**

Ask the questions below in any order:

> **And am I facing the right direction?**
>
> **And am I the right distance away?**
>
> **And am I at the right angle?**
>
> **And are you facing the right direction?**
>
> **And are you at the right distance?**
>
> **And are you at the right angle?**

It's just that simple.

Here is a blending example that is a bit more complicated. We will pick up where I start to deviate from the Clean Space start.

Example #3: Clean Space...Clean Spinning...Clean Language

My client Ellie is working outside, doing a Clean Space session. She has identified six spaces that hold various bits of information about the romantic relationship she has chosen to explore. She is back now at Space #4.

Clean Space in progress...

Facilitator: **And return to** Relationship. **And what do you know...from there...about** Stay or Go? (gesturing toward Space #5)

Ellie: *I know that when I look at it, I feel anxious, but if I'm not looking at it, then I'm okay.*

Since Ellie has described feeling different when she looks at the space or looks away, I decide to have her explore more about the "not looking at" experience by asking a set of Clean Spinning questions.

Facilitator: **And turn in either direction...until it seems right to stop.**

Ellie makes a quarter turn so that her right shoulder is toward Space #5.

Facilitator: **And what do you know...from there?**

Ellie: *I know that there is more to my life than that one relationship. If I look out this way, I see that.*

Facilitator: **And turn again in either direction...until it seems right to stop.**

Again Ellie makes a quarter turn.

Facilitator: **And what do you know...from there?**

Ellie: *I know that with some distance, I feel calmer. I can consider what I want better. It's not such a desperate want.*

I hear Ellie describe her want as if it has personal qualities: *it* is not so desperate. So I invite her to notice a bit more about *it*.

Facilitator: **And what kind of** a want **is that** want?

Ellie: *It's a want like planning for a trip, deciding what you want to take, deciding where you want to go. It's a thoughtful and calm want, not one that rushes to grab an answer it can hold on to, like a life preserver.*

Facilitator: **And where is that** thoughtful, calm want**?**

Ellie: *It's just below my heart, and I can access that want if I think about that spot.*

Facilitator: **And what kind of** deciding **is that** deciding**?**

Ellie: *When the want is calm and thoughtful, then deciding is effortless.*

I have to decide in this moment whether I let this session become one focused on the metaphors or I stick more closely to Clean Spinning and Clean Space. Since I already have a good deal of information about six spaces, I decide to stay with the spatial work. The metaphor is now in Ellie's conscious awareness; it will be part of the session even if we move on. I return to Clean Spinning.

Facilitator: **And turn again in either direction...until it seems right to stop.**

Ellie turns a quarter turn and again finds some additional information to broaden her perspective. When I invite her to turn yet again, I am surprised when she doesn't continue her pattern of quarter turns. Evidently her subconscious has two more points to reveal, and she makes only a 45 degree turn. Again she discovers more information. I invite her to turn another time, and she returns to where she began, facing Space #5.

Facilitator: **And what do you know...from there?**

Ellie: *I know that I'm making this harder than it needs to be. I was just so hyper-focused on the relationship that I kept dissecting it, like I was seeing it under a microscope. I needed to step back and look around.*

I stop Clean Spinning at this point. It seems more relevant to me that Ellie is back where she began, that she has turned five times and not six. I return to Clean Space. Ellie has so much new information from spinning in this space that I decide to check in to see whether the name of the space has changed.

Facilitator: **And what could this space be called now?**

Ellie: *It definitely feels different! It's...not so different and yet it's all different. It's called "Relationships."*

And Ellie adds an *s* to the word Relationship on the post-it.

Facilitator: **And what do you know from** Relationships **now...about** Stay or Go?

Ellie: *I do know what I want. Now it's a matter of figuring out timing, but I know... I know.*

So you see how it might go if you blend questions from one or more of the processes with another. I made my choices based on what my client said. I judiciously selected questions from a few other Clean processes to insert into what was basically a Clean Space session.

This kind of blending skill becomes natural once you are very familiar and comfortable with the various processes individually. I do not recommend playing around with this when you are learning. You need to be "off script," with the questions and processes automatic, before you have some leftover attention you can devote to the subtle nuances of a client's words and alternative, deliberate choices to be made in the moment.

Physicalizing the metaphors

Ready for a bigger challenge? Here's another spatial approach you can use, one that focuses on helping a client explore his metaphors. I select questions from many of the Clean processes we have covered, and you will see how I blend them.

I start by having my client complete a Before Our Session sheet, which includes a drawing that shows how what he wants would look. After exploring this a bit with Clean Language questions, I will invite him to re-create his drawing in the space available, whether it is indoors or outdoors, using whatever is at hand. Like drawing, it is a way of *physicalizing the metaphors*. My questions will then guide my client to move about in this metaphor landscape, discovering more about the metaphors and what he knows from the various spaces on which he stands.

Remember: to have a clean intention means it is not my goal to make anything happen, to fix anything. I simply want to guide my client's attention and exploration in ways that build on what is emerging for him, trusting that his mind/body system will learn from itself what it needs to know at this time.

To give you an idea of what I will be drawing from, here is a list of most of the questions/directives I will be using in this next session.

From Clean Language and Before Our Session sheet

"**And what would you like to have happen?**"

"**And what kind of [x] is that [x]?**"

"**And is there anything else about that [x]?**"

"**And where is that [x]?**"

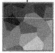

From Clean Space

> "And find a space where you are in relation to that [x]…now."

> "And find a space that knows something about [x]."

> "And what do you know…from there?"

> "And what do you know…now?"

> "And what difference…does knowing that…make?"

From Clean Boundaries

Just because David Grove developed Clean Boundaries to work with a client's drawing doesn't mean you cannot adapt it for when your client locates his metaphors in actual, physical spaces if he mentions a boundary of some sort. Rather than drawing new boundaries on a piece of paper, you can use the same Clean questions and have your client mark expanding boundaries with post-its or whatever other props the client chooses. If you are working outside, paper blows away easily, so sticks, stones, bricks, pieces of rope, cones, etc., usually work better.

> "And where does that space go?"

> "And what kind of boundary does that space have?"

> "And what kind of space is beyond that boundary?"

From Clean Action

> "And how will you [x]?"

> "And when will you [x]?"

From Clean Closures

"And as we're just about out of time, I invite you to find out what happens when [x]."
"And would this be a good place to stop for right now?"

Watch for how I blend and weave questions from the different processes we have covered to respond to what comes up for my client. This session is being conducted outside, in a garden. People often make meaning out of all sorts of available material, and the outdoors offers plenty, some static (bodies of water, paths, gates, flowers, etc.) and some moving (clouds, wind, birds flying, etc.). If you have the option to be outside, I encourage you to experiment!

Example #4: Clean Language and Before Our Session sheet...
Clean Space...Clean Boundaries...Clean Action...Clean Closures

Matt's Before Our Session sheet:

What would you like to have happen?

I want to nourish myself better.

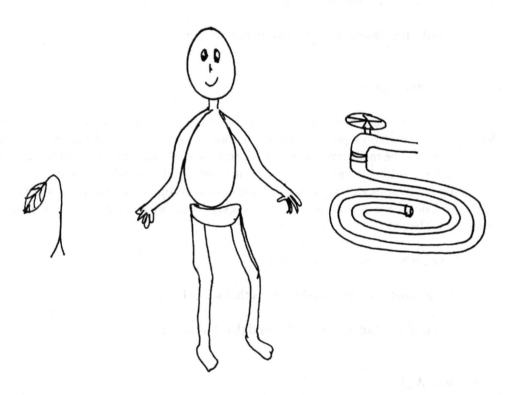

Even if my client has already written an answer, I ask this next question so that his exact words are spoken aloud and to give him another chance to change or add to them after having done the drawing, which might have revealed more information.

Facilitator: **And what would you like to have happen?** (gesturing toward the drawing)

Matt: *I want to nourish myself better.*

Looking at his drawing, I can't tell whether Matt is the figure by the spigot and hose (the *I*) or he is the plant (the *myself*). Sounds like it. Perhaps differentiating these selves will be helpful for him. I start with a few clarifying Clean Language questions before having him physicalize what is on the page, easing into it with a conversational Clean question (more about this on pages 184–185).

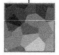

Facilitator:	**And would you like to describe your drawing?**

Matt:	*That's me…And here's the spigot. And that small, droopy plant is me too, somehow. Huh…I didn't realize that when I drew it.*

Facilitator:	**And a** small, droopy plant is you too. **And is there anything else about that** plant?

Matt:	*It's a little package of potential. It just needs the right kind of nourishment, all the right components, to be in the perfect growing environment. But I don't know what that is or where to get it.*

Facilitator:	**And a** little package of potential. **And what kind of** potential **is that** potential?

Matt:	*Well, it can't be anything it wants to be, because it is, after all, this type of plant. Actually, I think it's a kind of tree! It can grow as big as this kind of tree grows, it can spread out, it can produce food for creatures. Maybe it can protect others. It could potentially do all kinds of things. And it doesn't have to decide or choose now. It just needs to grow healthy, getting what it needs for now.*

There is one more element of Matt's drawing he has yet to mention. I would like to find out his exact words for it and bring his attention to it before inviting him to physicalize his drawing.

Facilitator:	**And is there anything else about…that?** (gesturing to the hose in the drawing)

Matt:	*Yes, that's the hose that I can use to water the plant.*

Matt has expressed his want in metaphoric terms: the tree needs to grow healthy with the right kind of nourishment. He knows that there will be more than one component needed; already we see a spigot and a hose, suggesting there might also be water and a source of that water.

Clean Space is a good process to use when your client wants to discover and/or consider multiple options or components. I am going to consider "meeting the tree's needs" as the want, since Matt has identified himself as the *droopy plant*, and blend the structure of the Clean Space process with Clean Language.

Facilitator:	And would you be interested in exploring all this (gesturing to the drawing) in this space around us? (gesturing out and around)

Matt:	*Sure. I like trying different stuff.*

Facilitator: **And that** (gesturing to drawing) **would look like what?** (gesturing around the space)

After wondering around for awhile, Matt picks up a twig and sticks it in the ground in an open area of mulch.

Matt: *Here feels right. This is the tree, the droopy plant.*

Matt starts moving around the garden again and spots an actual hose bib. He looks back and forth between the hose bib and the twig, removes the twig, and replaces it in another place in the mulch, about 12 feet from the hose bib.

Facilitator: **And there?** (gesturing to the spigot)

Matt: *That's the spigot, and this* (marking a spot by drawing in the mulch with a stick) *is where the hose is.*

Facilitator: **And place yourself where you are in relation to that** (gesturing to tree)... **now.**

Matt settles himself about eight feet away from and sideways to the twig, with his right shoulder facing it. He looks up and nods. (We will call this Space #1.)

So the key metaphors in Matt's drawing have been located: himself, the plant, the hose, and the spigot.

Facilitator: **And what do you know...from there?**

Matt: *That the tree is out of my reach. And sort of out of my sight. It's in my peripheral vision, but it's easy not to notice it.*

I decide to use one of the optional Clean Space questions where the facilitator selects a specific word/phrase the client has said to ask about.

Facilitator: **And what do you know from there...about that spigot?**

Matt: *I know it works. I can see the other plants nearby look healthy and well watered.*

Facilitator: **And what do you know from there...about that hose?**

Matt: *It's connected, but it's not on.*

Facilitator: **And what do you know from there...about right kind of nourishment?**

Matt: *I know it's important, but it's sort of like out of sight, out of mind. I'm just assuming it's getting what it needs.*

Because this space is where Matt located his droopy tree—physicalizing his metaphor—I do not ask what it is called. Not that you couldn't; it might be interesting, but it's not a part of the Clean Space process I chose to blend into this session.

Now back to Matt. "*Getting what it needs*" sounds related to his original want, so I suggest a specific space to find. (Remember, this is an option you have in Clean Space—though it is definitely more directive than leaving the space the client finds entirely up to him.)

Facilitator: **And find a space that knows about** the right kind of nourishment.

Matt goes to stand by the hose bib, facing the twig.

Facilitator: **And what do you know…from there?**

Matt: *Well, I know I haven't turned on the water. Guess that's why the plant is so droopy. I get this strong feeling from here that it needs this water—almost like a thirsty feeling.*

Facilitator: **Find another space that knows something else about the** right kind of nourishment.

Matt moves to a space not far from Space #1 and looks down at his feet intently.

Facilitator: **And what do you know…from there?**

Matt: *I know I've sort of ignored this hose. It's so close to where I was standing, but I didn't even notice it. Huh…*

I am wondering how it is that these spaces are so close together and yet Matt has not been seeing the objects. He seems puzzled too, though what about I do not know exactly. I decide some Clean Boundaries questions might be useful as a way to further explore these spaces and how they relate to one another. So I return Matt to where he began.

Facilitator: **Return to** (gestures to Space #1). **And what kind of space is that space?**

Matt: *It's a closed-in sort of space, like it's a bubble. No, not a bubble really, more like…well, this is going to sound really weird, but it's sort of like an amniotic sack, but one where everything goes in to nourish it but nothing goes out.*

Facilitator: **And is there anything else about** nothing goes out?

Matt: *Yes, that doesn't feel right. Like, I can move around in it. It's like I've never known anything else, so it seems normal, but it's not normal.*

Facilitator: **And where does that space go?**

Matt: *Not far. Just beyond my outstretched arms.*

Facilitator:	**And what kind of boundary…does that space have?**
Matt:	*It's flexible; it gives if I push on it. And it's sort of transparent.*
Facilitator:	**And what kind of space…is beyond that boundary?**
Matt:	*It's where the hose is. It's open and airy and easy to move in* (pause). *And it's where the soil is.*

Because Matt made a point of adding this detail, I ask a Clean Language question about it.

Facilitator:	**And what kind of** soil **is that** soil?
Matt:	*It's rich soil, full of nutrients for growing plants.*
Facilitator:	**And where does that space go?**
Matt:	*It's deep. Deep enough for any tree roots. And it's always there, even if we can't see it, like under a building or something.*
Facilitator:	**And what kind of boundary…does that space have?**
Matt:	*It goes down to the bedrock.*
Facilitator:	**And what kind of space…is beyond that boundary?**
Matt:	*It's solid rock. And it goes a long way down. There's a permanence about it.*
Facilitator:	**And where does that space go?**
Matt:	*To the underground water table. There's water there! I kind of assumed the spigot would be connected to some municipal water supply, but no…it goes to a well fed by the underground water table.*

Because Matt's intention is to find nourishment for his plant and because, logically, plants need water, I add a Clean Language question here to explore this a bit more.

Facilitator:	**And is there anything else about that** underground water table?
Matt:	*I didn't realize it was there. Always running, flowing…always below the ground I stand on…always available to tap into.*

I generally pause for quite awhile when a client makes a discovery like this one. Matt often finds it very moving to connect with a resource that is "always there." Many will use words like *sacred*, *divine*, and *loving* in describing it. They usually close their eyes. I am panning for gold here, creating the conditions for an emergence process to unfold on its own, so I am not going to ask more questions about it. But I wait silently for awhile, and let Matt savor this feeling.

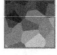

Matt's breathing shifts, and he seems ready to move on. I ask:

Facilitator: **And what kind of boundary…does that space have?**

Matt: *It's more like an energetic edge, a thin bubble membrane that separates the bedrock and soil and the underground water from the molten core of Earth below, and it goes above the Earth the same distance, into the air.*

Facilitator: **And what kind of space…is beyond that boundary?**

Matt: *It's limitless, atmospheric space.*

Facilitator: **And is there anything else about that space?**

Matt: *It's where the sun is!* (And he turns and lifts his face to the sun, eyes closed.)

Now, I have a choice, since I am blending processes. I could keep going out for more spaces and boundaries. I could start to go in reverse and ask what each space and boundary knows. Or I could abbreviate the process and jump back to where we started Clean Boundaries. I choose this last option because of where I decide Matt's attention would best be directed.

Look back at Matt's original statement. Notice he didn't say "I want to be better nourished." He said "*I want to better nourish myself.*" This implies that, at some level, he knows he is the one who wants or needs to deliver the nourishment. So given that our time is limited, I am going to help him explore now: what does *he* know about the nourishment and his role in it?

Facilitator: **Return to** (gesturing to Space #1). **And what do you know from there… now?**

Matt returns to his first spot, but this time he stands facing the twig directly.

Matt: *I thought the tree was out of my reach. Maybe because it was just in my pe ripheral vision, where it was easy not to notice it. But it is within my reach. I just have to move a little! I can move a little to reach the spigot. I can move a little to pick up the hose. I can turn to face the tree.*

Now Matt might do all this in his mind, but he doesn't. He walks to the hose bib and mimes turning it on. He walks to the imagined hose, mimes picking it up, faces the twig, and motions turning on the water from a hose nozzle. He returns to Space #1, standing silent, and I wait patiently until he seems finished processing. I repeat the question, as Matt may have new information.

Facilitator: **And what do you know from there…now?**

Matt: *I know I can water that droopy plant and revive it and help it grow.*

Here again, I return to Clean Language to hold Matt's attention on his role in this nourishment.

Facilitator:	**And** you *can* water that droopy plant. **And what kind of** you *can* water a droopy plant and revive it and help it grow**?**
Matt:	*It's an aware me that pays attention to what the plant needs.*
Facilitator:	**And where is that** aware…**when you** pay attention to what the plant needs**?**
Matt:	*It's in my heart.*
Facilitator:	**And is there anything else about that** heart that's aware**?**
Matt:	*The heart knows to use the amniotic fluid and the sun and the soil and the underground water to nourish the plant so the tree will grow.*
Facilitator:	**And what do you know now…about** nourish yourself better**?**
Matt:	*I know that I have to tune into my heart.*
Facilitator:	**And what difference…does knowing that…make?**
Matt:	*It makes all the difference. Before I was feeling sort of helpless, like the nourishment would just happen, would just come…or not. Like there wasn't anything I could do about it. Now I know what I can do. I can tune in to my heart!*

Now I pick up a few questions from the Clean Action process to help Matt take this new-found awareness into his life.

Facilitator:	**And** tune into your heart. **And how will you** tune into your heart**?**
Matt:	*I can meditate on this. It's not a problem; I know how to do this. I just needed to know what to be tuning in for.*
Facilitator:	**And when will you** meditate and tune into your heart**?**
Matt:	*I'll make it part of my morning ritual!*
Facilitator:	**And when will you start** making it part of your morning ritual**?**
Matt:	*Tomorrow.*

To wrap up, I pair up two Clean Closure options.

Facilitator:	**And as we're just about out of time, I invite you to find out what happens when** you meditate and tune into your heart…as part of your morning ritual…and be aware of what plant needs. **And would this be a good place to stop for right now?**
Matt:	*Yes, thank you!*

To blend or not to blend

So now you've found me out: I am not a purist when it comes to these processes. Truth be told, the example above is closest to the way I, personally, tend to conduct sessions: blending processes as I go. The questions and directives above are just some of the choices I might have made. If you had other ideas as you were reading along, they likely would have been effective too.

As you practice and master each process, you will get a clearer idea of what each helps your client accomplish in your particular context or with particular issues or types of clients. And once you are comfortable using many of these 12 processes, you can combine them in an endless variety of ways according to your own imagination, your intuition, your context, the time you have, and what your client says in the moment.

Spatial processes direct attention to the relationships between spaces and are a more externalized experience for the client, while CLQs can be directed to internalized metaphors. It is a delicate dance to work back and forth between the two successfully, and it means being very attuned to what is happening with your client.

Other Clean facilitators might disagree with me and argue strongly in favor of sticking to one process at a time. And I appreciate there is a case to be made in favor of that. If nothing else, the fewer choices the facilitator is making about where to direct attention, the Cleaner the facilitating is. "Trust the process, trust the client, and stay out of the way," you could well say.

I leave it to you to come to your own conclusions after you have been working with these Clean processes for awhile: to blend or not to blend.

INTEGRATING CLEAN PROCESSES

The third mix and match approach to using these Clean processes is to integrate them with other techniques and models of working with your clients. There is a continuum of ways to integrate Clean, from simply using Clean questions to "Clean up" another model's directives to applying whole Clean processes intact to another context.

The possibilities are endless, and a trip to London for the annual Clean Conference[11] will give you plenty of workshops to attend where you can hear about all the fascinating ways people around the globe are integrating Clean with other kinds of work. You can also explore Lawley and Tompkins's website[12] with its many articles on Clean applications from contributors around the world. And there is an ever-evolving online book[13] created by Sharon Small and Andrea Chiou that is a compilation of information supplied by people around the world as to how they are applying Clean Language.

I will give you a few examples of Clean being integrated with other approaches, but first, let me add a few cautionary words.

- Inserting some Clean questions into a model you already use is great. You will be surprised how powerful just asking a client or group members "What would you like to have happen?" can be. A well-placed "What kind of [x] is that [x]?" or "What do you know about [x] now?" can be very effective. Or simply repeat back a client's exact words; it seems so simple, so obvious, that you cannot imagine it can make a difference, but it can. Whether you are doing group therapy with domestic violence perpetrators or facilitating a yoga and meditation retreat, you can apply basic Clean principles and use some CLQs. You will not get a full appreciation for what Clean processes can do with this minimalist approach, but it may be just what you need in your context.

- There is a difference between adding some Clean questions to what you do (fine!) and adding some of what you do to a Clean session (not so good). David Grove spent years experimenting and refining the questions and processes he developed. It is awfully easy to start adding to one of his processes in well-intentioned ways and end up mucking it up. Over the years that Grove experimented with techniques and observed clients, he generally simplified and removed questions and directives from processes; he didn't add more. That should tell us something. It is not that there is never a place for a Clean-ish question, but it needs to be done very mindfully, and that comes once you have had lots of experience being Clean and really deeply knowing its intention and effect.

Conversational Clean questions

What if you are in a context where using the unusual syntax of CLQs will not be appropriate or somewhere you do not want to be encouraging a trance state? Maybe a classroom or board room or a meeting of colleagues. Can Clean still be useful? Can you subtly drop in a few CLQs? Absolutely!

Let's start by considering this next example, where the questioner's goal is to get his speaker to expand on what he is saying. What happens when the questioner uses "normal" language? (Now, I am exaggerating to make my point here; you might not regularly talk like this. But you will see how easily subtle word choices can have unintended effects.)

Example

Speaker: *I've noticed I'm drawn to the classes that challenge me to question.*

Questioner: Oh, that's interesting. Tell me more! I've never heard you describe it quite like that before. Can you elaborate on what intrigues you?

Notice the subtleties of these word choices:

Interesting suggests a cognitive assessment. Not only does it aim for the head, but it is about the questioner's head, about what *he* perceives as interesting!

Tell me more! The request is framed so that the emphasis is on asking the speaker to prepare an answer for the questioner rather than inviting self-exploration for the speaker's sake.

I've never heard puts the speaker's attention not only on the questioner but on the past. Part of the speaker's mind is directed to think about what he might have said in the past rather than on what he is saying and meaning now.

Elaborate and *intrigues* are not simple words; they require some extra mental/cognitive processing if only for brief moments.

The speaker did not use the word *intrigue.* He said *drawn to* and *challenge.* Those words subtly imply metaphors (and drawn to *like what*? Like a magnet? Like a marionette? Like watching a candle's flame?). Why substitute another word with its own implied meanings, associations, and assumptions?

It is so easy to have an intention to stay out of your client's content and process but subtly insert yourself.

So, what if you want to avoid the kind of problems the above example demonstrates but don't want to use classic CLQ phrasing?

Think Clean

You can "think Clean" as you encourage a speaker to learn more about what he means, to clarify his thoughts and expression of them.

- Keep your questions short; do not add a lot of filler. It just gives the speaker more to have to mentally process.

- Do not substitute what you *assume* is a synonym for the speaker's exact words. Ask about his exact words.

- Avoid referring to yourself. It distracts the speaker's attention from himself and his experience.

You can integrate Clean thinking by inserting simple adaptations of CLQs into your normal talking, making them more typically conversational. Dropping the trance-inducing word "And…," you could ask:

"Can you say more about that?"
"What's that like for you?"
"Is there anything else about that?"
"How do you want it to be?"
"What difference does that make?"

Compare this example of a conversational Clean question to the earlier one in the last example. Notice how it is short and simple and keeps the speaker focused on his own experience.

Speaker: *I've noticed I'm drawn to the classes that challenge me to question.*

Questioner: What sort of question?

There are few situations where you can't "Clean up" questions and responses to foster greater clarity and better communication.

INTEGRATING WITH OTHER PROCESSES OR METHODOLOGIES

There are many methodologies that lend themselves to integrating with Clean processes. Consider the following examples.

Art therapy

Art therapists provide a supportive, therapeutic environment for clients to express and explore themselves with paint, clay, or a myriad of other possible media. The images clients create are invariably metaphors for their personal experiences. What processes like Clean Start, Clean Language, Clean Hieroglyphics, and Clean Boundaries provide are structured ways for counselors and therapists to engage a client with the verbal and nonverbal material that emerges during his art making. *Without pulling the client out of his experience* to interpret or analyze, therapists can facilitate clients in deepening their exploration of their subconscious material and enhance the healing potential of their art making.[14]

Equine-assisted psychotherapy/equine-assisted learning

There are a number of equine therapy models in use. The EAGALA approach,[15] in particular, emphasizes metaphors. This equine therapy model keeps clients on the ground as horses move around in a field or arena. Clients are invited to *physicalize their metaphors*, using the horses as part of their metaphor landscape. Having moving metaphors that behave unpredictably adds a fascinating dimension to the therapy. Clean questions and processes lend themselves to helping the client's needs and solutions unfold as part of the experiential process without being subject to the therapist's or equine specialist's assumptions or worldview. Any number of the processes in this book, such as Clean Language and Before Our Session sheet, Clean Networks, Clean Space, and Clean Boundaries, can be applied. A blended process session, like Matt's in the garden (see pages 176–182), could easily translate to the field or arena.

Hypnosis/hypnotherapy

Grove called Clean Language "the natural language of trance."[16] The wording of CLQs, the repetition, the pacing, the using of a client's own words, the focusing of the client's attention on his inner experience…all work together to quickly and easily induce a mindful inner focus or trance state and connect with the subconscious.

Clean Language has deep roots in hypnosis. At one time, David Grove studied Ericksonian hypnosis intently. But he found he was "interested in a different structure of experience."[17] He moved away from the idea of the hypnotherapist providing the metaphors, the visual imagery, or his own hypnotic or posthypnotic suggestions. Grove became intrigued with how client-generated metaphors revealed his clients' internal experience. With sustained exploration and attention, a new level of awareness emerges, and clients' systems self-regulate and heal.

For the hypnotist or hypnotherapist who wants an easy way into his client's subconscious while keeping himself out of it, Clean offers both the tools (the CLQs) and the structure (the processes) to do so. Both invite intuitive responses that come from a place of deeper knowing.

Journal/poetry therapy

Repeatedly in this book I have advocated for the value of encouraging clients to process their "content" using a number of different media. Add writing to the list. It helps some clients sort out their thoughts, think them through more thoroughly, make connections, be expressive, and have a record to refer back to.

Journaling and writing poetry, with their inherent permission to creatively and intuitively explore one's inner world, have particular therapeutic benefits. The journal or poetry therapist can facilitate a session with Clean Language questions and/or other Clean processes and have clients respond to the experience in their journals or with poems. Or material from the journals or poems can be the starting point for a Clean process. As a certified facilitator of poetry therapy[18] techniques myself, I can attest to it: whichever comes first, they complement one another beautifully.

This is true for working with groups as well as individuals. Clean Metaphor Maps for Individuals in a Group Setting provides participants an experience to reflect by writing poetry or in their journals.

Sand tray therapy

Sand tray therapy uses a table of a specific dimension (so the whole of it can be seen without moving one's head) filled with sand. Typically, the therapist provides many small objects, such as wooden people and houses, that can be selected by the client. He is encouraged to create what in Clean Language facilitation, we would call a metaphor landscape, a representation of his world, experiences, and/or feelings. This book has introduced both Clean questions that could be selectively used and whole processes that integrate with this metaphor-based methodology. Clean Language questions, Clean Networks, Clean Space, or Clean Boundaries could all readily be used.

APPLICATIONS

Having established that you can simply drop in the occasional Clean question conversationally, use Clean processes individually or in sequence, and blend or integrate them with other methodologies, the question that remains is, what sorts of issues can be addressed with Clean? I think it is one of Clean's greatest strengths that the answer is, just about anything. Its use is not limited to any one issue or context. From trauma therapy to the classroom, from leadership development to stress management, with individuals or with groups, Clean processes can make a powerful difference.

I am constantly in awe of many contexts to which Clean facilitators apply their Clean skills. Here are a few examples. I will mention a couple of ways Clean might be used with each application, but these are by no means the only ways.

Addictions counseling

There is much that a person with a chronic addiction may not be willing to acknowledge, much he keeps below his conscious awareness, much that is painful or shameful to admit, even to himself. To avoid triggering subconscious defense mechanisms, counselors might consider those Clean processes that use metaphor. Start with Clean Language and metaphor maps. Perhaps they will segue into a Clean Hieroglyphics or Clean Boundaries session. They could lead to very surprising new perspectives for the addict in a way that does not feel confrontative or threatening.

Businesses/organizations

Clean is being used in many ways by businesses and organizations. It is becoming well known in Europe as an effective tool for encouraging creative and cohesive team work. Executive coaches use it to help leaders develop awareness of and improve their leadership styles and skills. Organizations elaborate their vision statements and strategic plans. Marketing teams use it to get inspiration; sales representatives and product developers determine what their customers *really* want. Working Cleanly can mean the right problems get addressed and collaborators better understand and communicate with one another.

These Clean processes are very different from the ways people in business are usually guided to work and reflect. In short order, people get engaged, which is helpful in and of itself. Even a brief Clean session can lead to profound insights and shifts.

Career counseling/coaching

Career counselors are expected to cover a lot of ground, providing information and building skills related to resume writing, job hunting techniques, interview strategies and skills, and more. Often though, clients come in with only a vague sense of what they want to do. Perhaps they want a change…or are forced to change…, but change to what? This needs to get sorted out if the time and energy the counselor and client invest are going to be well spent. Clean processes can help clients identify their values, interests, preferences, priorities, lifestyle concerns, and competing needs. Their insights can help them make appropriate choices.

And then there are the emotional issues related to job hunting. Whether it is a new grad anxious about getting his first job, a laid-off worker getting discouraged about ever getting hired again, or an at-home parent returning to work, clients often contend with feelings of inadequacy, pessimism, and frustration. Such feelings can undermine the best efforts of both career counselors and job seekers. Clean processes can reveal such underlying issues and help build internal resources.[19]

Working with physical symptoms

Just where does the mind stop and the body begin? The longer I work with clients, the fuzzier the boundary seems. Perhaps the two are simply inaccurate metaphors, suggesting a boundary that does not really exist. Mind and body are part of the same system, a self-organizing system.

Clean processes can be used in conjunction with appropriate medical care to address physical issues. For example, with symptoms that are the physical manifestations of inner issues like trauma, stress, anxiety, depression, and so on, exploring their subconscious roots in ways that lead to new perspectives and self-regulation strategies can help a client's entire system shift.

Health and wellness professionals from many disciplines can benefit from having Clean processes in their toolboxes to help address their clients' ills. Among my trainees have been a nurse, a doctor, an energy/body worker, a hospice chaplain, an acupuncturist, a shiatsu therapist, and a yoga teacher. Those whose scope of practice does not include treatment for mental health issues can particularly benefit from the lean methodologies in this book, as they make good assessment tools. Once the client presents a clearer picture of his key issues, the practitioner can use his other healing modality to address them.

School counseling

School counselors do not have the luxury of 50 minutes for a session/meeting. They are lucky to have 20 minutes with a student, parent, or teacher. They need processes that can get to the crux of the matter quickly, keep the discussion on track, and help the person coming for guidance get clear on what he wants or needs and/or formulate a plan of action. Clean Language and Before Our Session sheets (with or without a drawing) can quickly focus the discussion. Clean Action Space can be very effective for making a plan and is simple enough that students can learn to do it for themselves going forward.

Often school counselors work with groups. It might be an issue-based group (for example, anger management or grief and loss) or a class looking to improve its functioning as a team. Clean Metaphor Maps for Individuals in a Group Setting and Clean Group Metaphors can readily be adapted to the school context.

FINAL WORDS

One of the many beauties of these 12 Clean processes is how flexible they are and how readily they lend themselves to your creative applications with all sorts of different clients or client situations.

I hope you will find wonderfully inspiring and effective ways to use them. And when you do, I hope you will share them with the Clean community (see Resources on page 210) so we can all learn from one another and expand the use of this extraordinary work in the world.

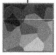

12 Lean Clean Processes Scripts

I have compiled all the scripts for the 12 lean Clean processes you have learned in the following pages where you can readily find them. I have also reduced each to only one page so you can copy and refer to it without shuffling papers when you are practicing facilitating. In some cases, fitting the script on a page means there are options detailed in the text that are not here. Once you get comfortable with the basics, check back with the text portion to see what else you might add. You will probably find it interesting to revisit the text after a few rounds anyway, as you may have questions. And the text is likely to have even more relevance for you once you have had some experience with clients with the process.

There is another advantage to having the scripts all here together: when you look over them in order, I think you will notice how easily they flow one into the next.

And finally, remember what I said at the start: the difference between reading a book like this and finding it a "stimulating read" and having it rock your world is in the doing!

CLEAN SITUATING

Step #1

"And where would you like to be?"

Step #2

"And where would you like me to be?"

CLEAN START

Where [x] is the post-it, drawing, or object that represents the client's topic or goal.

Step #1: Establishing the client's want or topic of inquiry

>**"And draw or write what you would like to have happen…or to know more about."**

>**"And choose an object to represent what you would like to have happen…or to know more about."**

Step #2: Setting up

>**"And place that** (gesturing to the paper/object) **where it seems…right."**

>**"And place yourself where you are in relation to that** (gesturing to the paper/object)**…now."**

Step #3: Aligning the spaces (ask about six of these questions, in any order)

>**"And are you in the right space?"**
>**"And is [x] in the right space?"**

>**"And are you at the right height?"**
>**"And is [x] at the right height?"**

>**"And are you facing the right direction?"**
>**"And is [x] facing the right direction?"**

>**"And are you at the right angle?"**
>**"And is [x] at the right angle?"**

>**"And are you at the right distance from [x]?"**
>**"And is [x] the right distance from you?"**

>**"And are you in the right position?"**
>**"And is [x] in the right position?"**

Step #4: Synthesizing

>**"And what do you know…from there?"**

Option: **"And is there anything else you know…from there?"**

BEFORE OUR SESSION

To have a focus to begin our session, please answer the following question. Feel free to write as little or as much as you like.

And what would you like to have happen?

Draw a sketch of what this would look like. NO artistic talent is required here; stick figures are fine. Use another paper or the back of this one if you need more room.

Section Two CLQs to develop more details about the above:

"**And** [client's word(s)]."
"**And what kind of** [x] **is that** [x]?"

"**And** [client's word(s)]."
"**And is there anything else about that** [x]?"

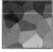

CLEAN SPINNING

Where [x] is the post-it, drawing, or object that represents the client's topic or goal.

Step #1: Establishing the client's want or topic of inquiry

> **"And draw or write what you would like to have happen…or to know more about."** (gesturing to the paper and markers)

> or

> **"And choose an object to represent what would you like to have happen…or to know more about."** (gesturing to objects or around the space)

Step #2: Setting up

> **"And place that where it seems…right."**

> **"And place yourself…where you are in relation to that…now."**

Step #3: Gathering information

> **"And what do you know…from there?"**

> **"And turn in either direction…until it seems right to stop."**

> **"And what do you know…from there?"**

Repeat about three to five more times:

> **"And turn again…until it seems right to stop."**

> **"And what do you know…from there?"**

Step #4: Synthesizing

As your client faces his goal (written, drawn, or object):

> **"And what do you know…now?"**

> **"And what difference…does knowing that…make?"**

CLEAN NETWORKS

Where [x] is the post-it, drawing, or object that represents the client's topic or goal.

Step #1: Establishing the client's want or topic of inquiry

> **"And draw or write what you would like to have happen…or to know more about."** (gesturing to the paper and markers)

> or

> **"And choose an object to represent what would you like to have happen…or to know more about."** (gesturing to objects or around the space)

Step #2: Setting up

> **"And place that** (gesturing to the paper/object) **where it seems…right."**

> **"And place yourself where you are in relation to that** (gesturing to the paper/object)**…now."**

Step #3: Gathering information

> **"And what do you know…from there?"**

Repeat about five times:

> **"And find another space."** (gesturing all around)

> **"And what do you know…from there?"**

Step #4: Synthesizing

> **"And return to your first space."** (gesturing to the space)

> **"And what do you know from there…now?"**

> **"And what difference…does knowing that…make?"**

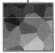

CLEAN NETWORKS: MOVING THE OBJECT

Step #1: Establishing the client's want or topic of inquiry

> **"And draw or write what you would like to have happen...or to know more about."** (gesturing to the paper and markers)

> or

> **"And choose an object to represent what would you like to have happen...or to know more about."**

Step #2: Setting up

> **"And place that** (gesturing to paper/object) **where it seems...right."**

> **"And place yourself where you are in relation to that** (gesturing to paper/object)**...now."**

> **"And what do you know...from there?"**

> **"And what does that** (gesturing to paper/object) **know...from there?"**

Step #3: Gathering information

Repeat about five times:

> **"And find another space that** (gesturing to paper/object) **could go to."**

> **"And what does that** (gesturing to paper/object) **know...from there?"**

Step #4: Synthesizing

> **"And return that** (gesturing to paper/object) **to its first space."** (gesturing to the space)

> **"And return to your first space."** (gesturing to the space)

> **"And what do you know from there...now?"**

> **"And what difference...does knowing that...make?"**

CLEAN SPACE

Step #1: Establishing the client's want or topic of inquiry

> **"And draw or write what you would like to have happen…or to know more about."** (gesturing to the paper and markers)

> or

> **"And choose an object to represent what would you like to have happen…or to know more about."** (gesturing to object collection or around the space)

Step #2: Setting up

> **"And place that where it seems…right."** (gesturing to the paper/object)

> **"And place yourself where you are in relation to that** (gesturing to paper/object) **…now."**

Step #3: Gathering Information

> **"And what do you know…from there?"**

> **"And what do you know from there…about that?"** (gesturing to paper/object)

> **"And what could this space be called?"**

> **"And put that down."**

> **"And mark that space."** (gesturing to the space)

Locate 5 more spaces:

> **"And find another space."**

> **"And what do you know…from there?"**

> **"And what do you know from there…about that?"** (gesturing to the paper/object)

> **"And what could this space be called?"**

> If needed, add: **"And put that down"** and **"And mark that space."**

Step #4: Networking

"And return to [name of a space]**."** (gesturing toward the space)

"And what do you know from there...now?"

"And what do you know from there... about [name of another space]**?"** (gesturing toward the space)

Step #5: Synthesizing

"Return to [name of Space #1]**."** (gesturing toward the space)

"And when all that (all-inclusive sweeping gesture)**, what do you know...now?"**

"And what do you know now...about [x]**?"** (gesturing to goal/topic)

"And what difference...does knowing that (all-inclusive sweeping gesture)**... make?"**

CLEAN LANGUAGE QUESTIONS WITH METAPHOR MAPS

Step #1: Establishing topic/goal and drawing

> **"And what would you like to have happen?"**

> **"And that would look like what?"** (gesturing to paper and markers)

Step #2: Gathering information (where [x] is a word or phrase the client uses)

> **"And is there anything else about that [x]?"**

> **"And what kind of [x] is that [x]?"**

> **"And where is that [x]?"**

Step #3: Getting a new metaphor

> **"And that's [x]…like…what?"**

Adding new information to a drawing

> **"And that would look like what?"**

CLEAN HIEROGLYPHICS

Asked about written words on a starting paper or metaphor map:

Step #1: Gathering information (gesturing to the paper as you ask)

> **"And what do you notice…about the letters… or words?"**

> **"And what do you notice…about the spaces between the letters… or words?"**

> **"And what do you notice…about the placement of those letters… or words?"**

Prompt to add info to drawing:

> **"And that would look like what?"**

Gathering further details:

> **"And is there anything else…about that** [letter/word/space/] **placement?"**

> **"And what do you notice…about any other letters…or words…or spaces…or placement?"**

> **"And is there anything else you notice….about what's there?"**

> **"And what does that** [letter/word/space] **know?"**

Where [x] is your client's word(s):

> **"And is there anything else…about that** [x]**?"**

> **"And what kind of** [x]**…is that** [x]**?"**

Step #2: Synthesizing

> **"And what do you know…now?"** (gesturing to the whole paper)

> **"And what do you know now…about** [client's original topic/goal]**?"**

> **"And what difference…does knowing that…make?"**

CLEAN BOUNDARIES

Step #1: Setting up

Noticing a written or drawn boundary or edge. Explore what's within and the boundary itself—including words, lines, and symbols.

> **"And is there anything else…about that?"** (gesturing to words/objects)

> **"And what's that?"** (gesturing to objects, lines, boundaries, etc.)

Step #2: Gathering information

> **"And what kind of space…is beyond that boundary?"**

> **"And where does that space go?"**

> **"And what kind of boundary…does that space have?"**

Prompt to add info to drawing:

> "And that would look like what?"

Optional: You can ask for more details—but not every time.

> **"And is there anything else…about there/that?"** (gesturing to a space or boundary)

Step #3: Reversing direction

> **"And what does that boundary know?"**

> **"And what does that space know?"**

Continue on until you reach the original written statement:

> **"And what do that/those** [word(s)/symbol(s)] **know?"**

Step #4: Synthesizing

> "And what do you know…now?" (gesturing to the whole paper)

> "And what do you know now…about [client's original topic/goal]?"

> "And what difference…does knowing that…make?"

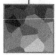

CLEAN ACTION

Step #1: Establishing a goal [x]

"And what would you like to have happen?"

Step #2: Gathering information

First action:

"And what's an action you know you can do...to [x]?"

"And how will you do that?" (repeat if necessary to get specifics)

"And when will you do that? (repeat if necessary to get specifics)

About five more actions:

"And what's another action you know you can do...to [x]?"

"And how will you do that?" (repeat if necessary)

"And when will you do that? (repeat if necessary)

Step #3: Synthesizing

"And what do you know...now?"

"And what difference...does knowing that...make?"

Options

"And is there anything else about that action...you know you can do?"

"And is there anything else about how/when**...you will do that?"**

CLEAN ACTION SPACE

Step #1: Establishing a goal [x]

> **"And draw or write what you would like to have happen."** (gesturing to paper and markers)

> or

> **"And choose an object to represent what would you like to have happen."**

Step #2: Setting up

> **"And put that** (gesturing to paper/object) **where it seems…right."**

Step #3: Gathering information

First action:

> **"And find a space that knows about an action you can to do…to [x]."**

> **"And from there…what do you know you can do…to [x]?"** (gesture to paper or object)

> **"And how will you do that?"** (Repeat until action(s) is/are quite specific.)

> **"And when will you do that?"** (Repeat until answer is specific.)

Ask for about five more actions:

> **"And find a space that knows about another action you can do…to [x]."**

> **"And from there…what do you know you can do…to [x]?"** (gesture to paper or object)

> **"And how will you do that?"** (Repeat until action(s) is/are quite specific.)

> **"And when will you do that?"** (Repeat until answer is specific.)

Step #4: Synthesizing

> **"And find a space that knows…about all this."** (gesturing to all the spaces)

> **"And from there…what do you know…now?"**

> **"And what difference…does knowing that…make?"**

OPTIONAL CLOSINGS

1. **"Take all the time you need over the next days or weeks to…**

   (adjust your wording to what was said in the session)

   > **…get more familiar with [x]."**
   > **…notice more about [x]."**
   > **…see what happens next."**

2. **"And, as we're just about out of time,…is there anything else about all that…for right now?"**

3. **"And would this be a good place to stop…for right now?"**

Write your own clean closing:

CLEAN METAPHOR MAPS FOR INDIVIDUALS IN A GROUP SETTING

Step #1: Establishing the clients' wants or topics of inquiry [x]

Each person completes a Before Our Session sheet, answering:

> **"And what would you like to have happen?"**

> **"And when that's what you would like to have happen, that would look like what?"**

Step #2: Gathering information

> **"And as you look at what that would look like…, what are you drawn to?"**

> **"And what do you know…about that?"**

> **"And that would look like what?"** (gesturing to draw/write on paper)

> **"And what else do you know…about that?"**

> **"And that would look like what?"** (gesturing to draw/write on paper)

Repeat three to five times.

> **"And looking at that drawing again…, what are you drawn to?"**

> **"And what do you know…about that?"**

> **"And that would look like what?"** (gesturing to draw/write on paper)

> **"And what else do you know…about that?"**

> **"And that would look like what?"** (gesturing to draw/write on paper)

Step #3: Synthesizing

> **"And what do you know…now?"** (gesturing to paper)

> **"And what difference…does knowing that…make?"**

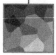

CLEAN GROUP METAPHORS

Step #1: Establishing the clients' goal [x]

> **"And what would you like to have happen?"**

Step #2: Creating a metaphor map

> **"And [x] would look like what?"**

Step #3: Present to group

Each participant presents his metaphor map. Another participants asks about some exact word or phrase [y] the participant uses or simply gestures to [y] on the page.

> **"And what kind of [y] is that [y]?"**

> **"And is there anything else about that [y]?"**

Step #4: Merging metaphor maps

Everyone has at least one contribution included in a new metaphor map.

Step #5: Merging group metaphor maps

Repeat Steps #3 and #4, having the larger groups present to each other, merge their ideas into a new metaphor map, and present to the next group.

Step #6: Synthesizing

With a single metaphor map, the facilitator reviews the description using the exact words of the participants and then asks these CLQs:

> **"And what do you know...now?"**

> **"And what do you know now...about [x]?"**

> **"And what difference...does knowing that...make?"**

What's Next?

BOOKS BY GINA CAMPBELL

If you are impressed by the powerful results you have gotten with clients using the Clean processes in this book and you are eager to learn more, I invite you to dive into Clean Language more deeply and specifically the Clean questions and strategies of Symbolic Modeling that focus on working with metaphors. My two books on the basics are workbooks: they take you step by step, with explanations, examples, and activities to practice, just as I do in trainings.

Mining Your Client's Metaphors: A How-To Workbook on Clean Language and Symbolic Modeling Basics Part One: Facilitating Clarity gives you the tools to help your clients learn more about their internal worlds and selves by exploring their inner metaphors.

Most people who come to helping and healing professionals want not just clarity but also some kind of change. *Mining Your Client's Metaphors: A How-To Workbook on Clean Language and Symbolic Modeling Basics Part Two: Facilitating Change* takes what you learn in Part One to even greater depths and then teaches you how to work with the metaphors of a client who wants change.

Both can be purchased from online retailers like Amazon and Barnes & Noble.

TRAINING

My in-person trainings use this book and the two described above as texts for the courses so you can spend less time taking comprehensive notes and more time getting lots of experience as both a facilitator and a client. Train with a group, and you will get helpful facilitation tips and lots of coaching and feedback as you progress.

Visit my website at www.miningyourmetaphors.com for details. You can sign up there for my newsletter to keep up to date on training events. Workshop events held at various conferences and other sites will be listed. Nothing coming up in the near future? Contact me and let me know your interest.

CERTIFICATION

Visit www.miningyourmetaphors.com for details about earning a certificate as a Clean Language Facilitator (CLF) or a Clean Spatial Facilitator (CSF). The program currently requires in-person courses, post-session supervision/coaching with practice clients, and the demonstration of competency with basic facilitation.

Resources

ON THE INTERNET

You can learn a lot about Clean Language, Symbolic Modeling, and what other people around the world are doing with Clean by visiting Penny Tompkins and James Lawley's website at www.cleanlanguage.co.uk. It serves as a sort of unofficial international collecting place for the Clean community. There, you will find literally hundreds of articles about Clean.

Mining Your Metaphor newsletter: visit www.miningyourmetaphors.com and sign up for Gina Campbell's newsletter, which will keep you notified of training opportunities, new publications, and other related topics.

Sharon Small and Andrea Chiou have created *Who Is Using Clean Language Anyway? A Compilation of Interviews of People Around the World Using Clean Language in Their Work.* The book is online and will continue to be added to as more Clean users submit their information. It will give you insight into the breadth of Clean's uses. Go to www.leanpub.com/whoisusingclean.

Sign up on Facebook for the group Clean Language Private Discussions (moderator: Brian Birch). There is an ongoing discussion of all things Clean and metaphor-related articles.

LinkedIn: Clean Language and Symbolic Modeling Research Group invites researchers interested in using Clean questions in their interviewing processes to share thoughts, questions, and information.

BOOKS ON *LEAN* CLEAN TOPICS

While there are a growing number of books about Clean Language and its derivatives, the books about what I call lean Clean processes, those that are relatively short and simple to facilitate, follow:

Cooper, Lynne & Castellino, Marietta (2012). *The Five-Minute Coach: Improve Performance Rapidly.* Carmarthen, Wales: Crown House Publishing.

Harland, Philip (2009). *The Power of Six: A Six Part Guide to Self-Knowledge.* London: Wayfinder Press.

OTHER BOOKS ON CLEAN TOPICS

Campbell, Gina (2012). *Mining Your Client's Metaphors: A How-To Workbook on Clean Language and Symbolic Modeling Basics Part One: Facilitating Clarity.* Bloomington, IN: Balboa Press.

Campbell, Gina (2013). *Your Client's Metaphors: A How-To Workbook on Clean Language and Symbolic Modeling Basics Part Two: Facilitating Change.* Bloomington, IN: Balboa Press.

Grove, David & Panzer, B. I. (1989). *Resolving Traumatic Memories: Metaphors and Symbols in Psychotherapy.* New York: Irvington Publishers, Inc.

Note the early date of this book. This is an interesting, if very dense, read, but be aware that Grove's work evolved considerably over the remaining two decades of his life. Out of print.

Harland, Philip (2012). *Trust Me, I'm the Patient: Clean Language, Metaphor, and the New Psychology of Change.* London: Wayfinder Press.

Lawley, James & Tompkins, Penny (2000). *Metaphors in Mind: Transformation through Symbolic Modelling.* London: Crown House Pub. Ltd.

Sullivan, Wendy, Meyer, Margaret, & Tosey, Paul (2015). *Clean Language in Business: 25 Applications of Metaphor at Work.* London: Crown House Publishing.

Sullivan, Wendy & Rees, Judy (2008). *Clean Language: Revealing Metaphors and Opening Minds.* Carmarthen, Wales: Crown House Publishing.

Walker, Caitlin (2014). *From Contempt to Curiosity: Creating the Conditions for Groups to Col-laborate Using Clean Language and Systemic Modelling.* Hampshire, England: Clean Publishing.

Way, Marian (2013). *Clean Approaches for Coaches: How to Create Conditions for Change Using Clean Language & Symbolic Modelling.* Hampshire, England: Clean Publishing.

Glossary of Terms

bottom-up approach/technique: a counseling or coaching strategy that makes no assumptions (or as few as humanly possible) and applies no categories. Its intent is to encourage open-ended exploration. A view of the client's system emerges from the details and their relationships.

Clean: refers to when a facilitator uses primarily a client's *exact* words and gestures and adheres to the inherent logic of his metaphors. Thus, a Clean question uses only a bare-bones structure of words that are the client's, and "staying Clean" means the facilitator offers no advice, interpretations, or alternative perspectives.

Clean Language: the special questions and syntax originally developed by counseling psychologist David Grove to encourage clients to explore their metaphors and inner worlds to better know themselves.

CLQ: stands for Clean Language question

co-inspiring object: David Grove's term for an object the client selects to represent his want or topic of inquiry. As a metaphor itself, it contributes its attributes and the associations a client has with it to his landscape.

downward causation: an aspect of the emergence process whereby the original component parts that made up the individual before a change are affected in turn. They change because the individual's system has a feedback loop: it learns from itself.

dream logic: Gina Campbell's term for a client's metaphor landscape's inherent logic. It may have its own rules of cause and effect, physics, time, space, etc., that are not consistent with everyday reality. It is more like what often happens in dreams: things suddenly appear and disappear, people morph into other people, animals talk, people fly...anything can happen!

embedded metaphors: words that suggest an image, object, or comparison not immediately noticeable to most people. Words that may have originally been easily spotted as metaphors have become so familiar that we easily overlook their references to other experiences. Examples: She *noted* the cap he had on. It's *beyond* comprehension.

emergence: a scientific concept that seeks to explain how a mass of individual units that have no single organizer can become a functioning, self-correcting system. Explains how complex systems change using simple rules, repetition, and feedback.

gestural metaphors: metaphors suggested by body movements.

Grovian: refers to a process or concept exhibiting a fundamentally Clean approach as developed by David Grove.

Grovian hypnosis: a distinctive method involving tone, pacing, Clean Language questions, and the client's exact words to naturally induce a deeply mindful state, fostering connection with the client's subconscious mind.

internalized metaphors: largely subconscious metaphors that encode a client's experiences and his interpretations of them. Also referred to as *personal* or *inner metaphors.*

invitation to metaphor: the facilitator asks a Clean Language question that asks for a metaphor for a feeling, gesture, experience, etc., that a client introduces (CLQ: "And that's *like* what?"). In these lean processes, a metaphor is generally sought for a resource or want.

logic of the landscape: refers to the idiosyncratic characteristics of a client's metaphors and their interactions. Each client's landscape of metaphors has its own rules and processes, which may or may not coincide with our daily, earthly logic (for example, if a heart is surrounded in ice, heat may melt the ice...or simple awareness of the ice or a vibration could melt it, etc.). Whatever rules the client's description establishes, for the facilitator to stay true to the "logic of the landscape" means his questions adhere to those rules.

metaphor: A figure of speech where one thing is equated to a decidedly different thing to clarify the nature of the first thing's traits or qualities. Metaphors are often used to describe abstract concepts and emotions. Grove uses the term "metaphor" broadly; he included similes, analogies, parables, and the like.

metaphor landscape: the sum total of a client's symbolic images as they relate to one another.

metaphor map: a client's depiction of his metaphors as they relate spatially to one another, like locations on a map.

modeling: the process of developing a model of the client's internal world (which may include his internalized metaphors) and the way his system is organized and functions. Modeling by the facilitator entails using a variety of strategies to help a client discover and experience his symbols and their interactive relationships and patterns.

natural trance: a hypnotic state induced by conversational guidance (as compared to a formal, scripted induction). A deeply self-reflective state; a state of mindful inner focus with easier access to the subconscious. Clean Language facilitation frequently induces a natural trance state in a client.

neuroplasticity: the brain's capacity to be flexible, to change, to grow new neurons and new connections between neurons.

physicalizing metaphors: refers to putting a metaphor into some kind of physical form. Examples: a drawing, a clay model, or using props in a room or outdoor area.

psychoactive space: a term coined by David Grove to describe a place or space filled with information from the client's inner experience with which he actively engages.

resource: that which a client identifies as being helpful or of some value to him. It could be a tool, person, skill, knowledge, place, feeling, attitude, etc. It is context specific.

resource state: a *feeling* or *state of being* that once achieved, will help a client do what he wants to do or change what he needs to change.

resource symbol: a symbol or metaphor that is helpful to a client in some way.

self-modeling: when a client explores his inner world for himself, discovering new information about its elements and/or metaphors and their relationships and patterns. Clients engage in self-modeling in every Clean session.

symbolic domain: A client is described as being "in his symbolic domain" when he is in an inner-focused, mindful state, exploring and experiencing his internalized metaphors. We say he "leaves the symbolic domain" when he returns to an alert, fully conscious awareness of his surroundings; he is no longer in touch with his metaphors in an *experiential* way.

Symbolic Modeling: a language-based, mind/body process that invites a client to achieve greater clarity about any personal topic, including himself, and to work through problematic issues at a very deep level. It uses three elements: Clean Language, metaphors, and modeling. Developed by James Lawley and Penny Tompkins, based primarily on David Grove's Clean Language work.

systems thinking: approaching a whole (such as a person or organization) as an interactive system of parts. In linear thinking, the emphasis is on how one part influences another part (cause and effect). Systems thinking pays particular attention to the feedback the effecting part gets and how it responds in turn.

top-down approach/technique: a counseling or coaching strategy based on a model that has established categories, types, or scripted exercises. The counselor or coach is guided as to how to work with the client based on a theory as to what best suits that type of client or situation. Examples: Myers-Briggs Inventory and Enneagrams.

Bibliography

Campbell, Gina (2012). *Mining Your Client's Metaphors: A How-To Workbook on Clean Language and Symbolic Modeling Basics Part One: Facilitating Clarity.* Bloomington, IN: Balboa Press.

Campbell, Gina (2013). *Your Client's Metaphors: A How-To Workbook on Clean Language and Symbolic Modeling Basics Part Two: Facilitating Change.* Bloomington, IN: Balboa Press.

Grove, David (11/13/1998). *The Philosophy and Principles of Clean Language.* www.clean-language.co.uk.

Grove, David with Wilson, Carol (2005). *Emergent Knowledge (EK) and Clean Coaching: New Theories of David Grove.* First published in *The Model* (British Board of NLP magazine). Available on www.cleanlanguage.co.uk/articles.

Harland, Philip (2009). *The Powers of Six: A Six Part Guide to Self-Knowledge.* London: Wayfinder Press.

Lakoff, George & Johnson, Mark (1980). *Metaphors We Live By.* Chicago: University of Chicago Press.

Lawley, James & Tompkins, Penny (2000). *Metaphors in Mind: Transformation through Symbolic Modelling.* London: Crown House Pub. Ltd.

Lawley, James & Tompkins, Penny (2002). *What Is Emergence?* www.cleanlanguage.co.uk.

Lawley, James & Tompkins, Penny (2003). *Clean Space: Modeling Human Perception through Emergence.* www.cleanlanguage.co.uk.

Lawley, James & Tompkins, Penny (2009). *Clean Space Revisited.* www.cleanlanguage.co.uk.

Rodgers, T., Milkman, K., John, L., & Norton, M. *Making the Best Laid Plans Better: How Plan-Making Increases Follow-Through.* http://scholar.harvard.edu/files.

Seigel, Daniel J. (2011). *Mindsight: The New Science of Personal Transformation.* New York: Bantam Books

Walker, Caitlin (2014). *From Contempt to Curiosity: Creating the Conditions for Groups to Collaborate Using Clean Language and Systemic Modelling.* Hampshire, England: Clean Publishing.

Endnotes

[1]*Mining Your Client's Metaphors: A How-To Workbook on Clean Language and Symbolic Modeling.* The two workbooks in this series teach a process based on David Grove's extraordinary work with metaphors (Clean Language) and further developments by James Lawley and Penny Tompkins (Lawley & Tompkins, 2000). My workbooks teach skills about how to go deeply into a person's inner world and use strategies for how to work with the metaphors the client finds there to nurture clarity, growth, and healing.

[2]Besides the articles in Resources that relate emergence to Clean Language specifically, a quick Internet search on the science of emergence will give you plenty of suggestions for where you can read more. For a layman's-style read, try *Emergence: The Connected Lives of Ants, Brains, Cities, and Software*, by Steven Johnson (2002). If you have a science/math background, *Signs of Life: How Complexity Pervades Biology*, by Richard Sole and Brian Goodwin (2002) would likely be more satisfying. For those interested in therapeutic applications, you might want to read *Chaos and Complexity: Implications for Psychological Theory and Practice*, by Michel R. Butz (1997).

[3]Tompkins, P. & Lawley, J. (1996). *And...what kind of man is David Grove? Rapport* magazine, Issue 33. Can be found at www.cleanlanguage.co.uk.

[4]Ibid.

[5]Ibid.

[6]You will find different writers about Clean Space may have slight variations as to the wording of the directives. I first learned Clean Space from Lawley and Tompkins in 2003, when they had spent some two years observing Grove's demonstrations with clients and developing a model of the process. Some of the changes Lawley and Tompkins have developed since then (Lawley & Tompkins, 2009) I have adopted; in other instances, I have kept some of the older ways. And I have made adjustments after studying Grove's Emergent Knowledge techniques with Angela Dunbar, also a Clean trainer, including changing the initial directive from "And put that where it needs to be" to "And put that where it seems right." Trying to be absolutely as Clean as possible is challenging, and both these phrasings have their issues with nuance. The best we can do as Clean facilitators is be as aware as possible of these nuances, observe how our clients respond to the Clean questions and directives, and make carefully considered decisions as to how to phrase them.

[7]Predating Grove's Clean Boundaries as a scripted process, Lawley and Tompkins, developers of Symbolic Modeling, described in their book what they called "broadening attention" beyond an implied boundary in the client's landscape. They also mention Grove's strategy of having the client add paper to the edges of his metaphor map if something on the paper (like a road) appeared to continue off the edge. For further details, see James Lawley and Penny Tompkins (2000), *Metaphors in Mind: Transformation through Symbolic Modelling*, London: Crown House Publishing Ltd., pp. 196–199.

[8]Rodgers, T., Milkman, K., John, L., & Norton, M. *Making the Best Laid Plans Better: How Plan-Making Increases Follow-Through.* http://scholar.harvard.edu/files._

[9]Ibid.

[10]Explore Penny Tompkins and James Lawley's website www.cleanlanguage.co.uk under Applications for some descriptions of group applications. For example, James's article *Metaphors of Organisation Part 2* describes some work with corporate clients.

[11]Visit Wendy Sullivan's site, www.cleanchange.co.uk, to find out more about the conference.

[12]Visit Lawley and Tompkins's website at www.cleanlanguage.co.uk/articles.

[13]Small, Sharon & Chiou, Andrea (begun 2014). *Who Is Using Clean Language Anyway? A Compilation of Interviews of People Around the World Using Clean Language in Their Work.* Find the e-book on www.leanpub.com/whoisusingclean.

[14]For deeper therapeutic work, I highly recommend Clean Language and Symbolic Modeling, which can also be applied to drawings. My two workbooks *Mining Your Client's Metaphors…* (see Resources) teach those skills.

[15]To learn more about EAGALA (Equine Assisted Growth and Learning Association), visit www.eagala.org.

[16]Op. cit., Tompkins, P. & Lawley, J. (1996).

[17]Ibid.

[18]Poetry therapy has been around as a field for over 30 years. To learn more about it visit www.poetrytherapy.org.

[19]For deeper therapeutic work, I highly recommend Clean Language and Symbolic Modeling. My two workbooks *Mining Your Client's Metaphors…* (see Resources on Clean topics) teach those skills.

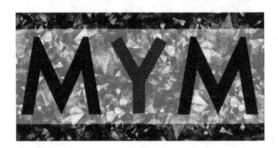

Printed in the United States
By Bookmasters